$14.95

NEW DEVELOPMENTS FOR MS SUFFERERS

BY APPOINTMENT ONLY SERIES
Arthritis, Rheumatism and Psoriasis
Asthma and Bronchitis
Cancer and Leukaemia
Heart and Blood Circulatory Problems
Migraine and Epilepsy
Do Miracles Exist?
Multiple Sclerosis
Neck and Back Problems
Realistic Weight Control
Skin Diseases
Stomach and Bowel Disorders
Traditional Home and Herbal Remedies
Viruses, Allergies and the Immune System

NATURE'S GIFT SERIES
Air – The Breath of Life
Body Energy
Food
Water – Healer or Poison?

WELL WOMAN SERIES
Menopause
Menstrual and Pre-Menstrual Tension
Pregnancy and Childbirth
Mother and Child

JAN DE VRIES HEALTHCARE SERIES
How to Live a Healthy Life
Questions and Answers on Family Health
The Five Senses
Inner Harmony
Healing in the 21st Century

THE JAN DE VRIES PHARMACY GUIDEBOOK SERIES
The Pharmacy Guide to Herbal Remedies

NATURE'S BEST SERIES
10 Golden Rules for Good Health

ALSO BY THE SAME AUTHOR
Life Without Arthritis – The Maori Way
Who's Next?

By Appointment Only series

New Developments for MS Sufferers

Jan de Vries

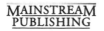
MAINSTREAM
PUBLISHING

EDINBURGH AND LONDON

First published in Great Britain in 2002 by
MAINSTREAM PUBLISHING COMPANY (EDINBURGH) LTD
7 Albany Street
Edinburgh EH1 3UG

ISBN 1 84018 464 7

A catalogue record for this book is available from the British Library

Typeset in Book Antiqua and Caslon
Printed and bound in Great Britain by
Cox & Wyman Ltd

Contents

Foreword to the 1985 Edition   7
Preface to the 1985 Edition   11
Preface to the 2002 Edition   15
Prologue   17
Chapter One Vitamins, Minerals and Trace Elements   49
Chapter Two Oil of Evening Primrose   53
Chapter Three Hyperbaric Oxygen   58
Chapter Four Acupuncture   63
Chapter Five Dental Care   68
Chapter Six Exercises, Drinking and Smoking   74
Chapter Seven Eating your Way to Better Health   83
Bibliography and Literature   141
Index   142

Foreword to the 1985 Edition

I find it uniquely pleasant to be connected with a book on methods of controlling Multiple Sclerosis. In 1950, I was solemnly informed, by no less a person than the President of the Multiple Sclerosis Society himself, that I should prepare for the end. My condition, in his opinion, was beyond hope. And a pitiable condition indeed it most certainly was. No one looking at me – unable to walk, to balance myself, to stand up, to see to any purpose, to talk clearly, to pick up a pen even, far less to write – would have questioned his opinion. But I am stubborn. And though others may have agreed with him (and who's to blame them?) I disagreed violently. I had my helpless carcass removed from the Queen Square Hospital by my loving wife and brought home. What happened then, I explain later. But before I leave you to read the book in peace, I have a few observations to make about its author.

Jan de Vries and I first met when he arranged that I should give a lecture in Amsterdam – with Jan himself translating it into Dutch – a language of which I am totally ignorant.

Then began an association which has lasted now for many years. It is based, I think, on a mutual respect. I respect him, for the breadth of his knowledge and his constant endeavour to widen it by studying different techniques in many different countries. He respects me, for reacting positively to the expert prediction of my imminent death, taking my future into my own hands, analysing my problem correctly and then solving it.

Our opinions meet in the realisation that there is no one and only way to control Multiple Sclerosis (or any other degenerative 'disease'), no one and only cause, no one and only way to help even one individual. Certain guidelines appear to be applicable to most people who are degeneratives. (Since we are all degenerating after a certain age – that being the price for living – I should perhaps refer to people who are degenerating too quickly.) I soon became aware that the regimen which had helped me, also helped a great variety of other people in that unfortunate category.

The fact that the correct diet helped not only Multiple Sclerosis sufferers, but also victims of other degenerative complaints, was first brought to my attention quite fortuitously.

A lady, who had put her husband on my regimen, rang up to say she wanted to come to London to visit me. As she intended to drive well over 100 miles, I tried to dissuade her, but she wouldn't listen. When she arrived the following day, it was to present me with a bottle of brandy and a huge basket of flowers, like the ones that stand beside film stars on gala occasions. I was completely taken aback. 'Don't tell me your husband has begun to improve already,' I said. 'It's not my husband,' she replied. 'It's me. My arthritis has gone completely.'

This is the story that emerged. Her husband had said the regime would be too horrible to follow. To encourage him to persevere, she joined him in following the diet strictly. And in the event her arthritis had vanished (physical problems clear up more quickly than do nerve problems).

What does this have to do with Jan de Vries? Not much, I suppose, except that it illustrates the sort of gratitude we both evoke from those we help. I can't speak for Jan, of course, but personally, over a period of many years, I have helped clear up almost every degenerative 'disease' in the book.

The case that is perhaps most outstanding is that of a composer, whom I first met in Santa Monica, Los Angeles. He was in hospital and on a breathing machine 24 hours a day. His problem was Amyotrophic Lateral Sclerosis, known there as Lou Gehrig's Disease, after a famous baseball player who died of it, and known in Britain also as Motor Neurone Disease.

I had been taken to see him by his sister, a screen-writing friend, who told me that he was in danger of being taken off his life support machine. Five doctors had met that morning, she told me, to decide on his future, and the vote had gone three to two against him. Quite understandably – there are queues of deserving cases waiting to be helped and he had had his time. His own doctor had argued so persuasively on his behalf that he had been granted a 'stay of execution'.

At that point I took over. He had money and was in a private room with a male nurse and also had his own fridge. I threw out the junk that was in there and stocked it with the appropriate foods. Then I had a long talk with his nurse.

A few months later, he was back home and on his machine only at nights. He acquired a secretary with a knowledge of music to whom he could dictate and began work again. Before I left America in 1982 he had already published two records of groups of songs. I had a letter a few years later telling me that he is still busily at work. Significantly too, since I last saw him he was hospitalised with pneumonia and came through unscathed.

Anyone who knows the customary course of this 'disease' – down and out in a year or so – will have to admit that something remarkable was achieved.

I report this case in detail, though I'm writing a foreword to a book by Jan de Vries. I know he has had many similar experiences, but they cannot carry conviction at second-hand. This is the sort of triumph that Jan has accomplished and he has done it time and time again. It is for Jan himself to tell you of them and to explain, in wiser language than mine, the various methods he has adopted.

Roger MacDougall

Preface to the 1985 Edition

In the early 1980s, I attended a lecture where a medical doctor spoke on the subject of Multiple Sclerosis. He stated that he could give 13 possible reasons for Multiple Sclerosis but that we have to compare this disease to an Agatha Christie thriller and find the answer to the mystery on the last page. However, he went on to say that the answer had not been found yet.

Listening attentively to him while he listed the 13 possible causes, I never heard him mention the word 'diet', which created the impression that Multiple Sclerosis as a degenerative disease and diet were not interconnected.

During question time, I asked him whether he thought that there was no connection between Multiple Sclerosis and diet. He replied that there was absolutely no relation, but that he had heard of people who stressed the importance of a dietary connection. These people, however, were only interested in making money out of this particular affliction. I could not help but inform him that when I studied acupuncture in China, I did not come across Multiple Sclerosis cases. Unfortunately, to my great surprise, visiting Taiwan a short time later to attend a congress in the city of Taipei, I was slightly surprised to be asked to give a lecture on this subject.

I asked the organisers on my arrival for the reason behind their choice of subject and was told that Multiple Sclerosis used not to be a problem there but, unfortunately, nowadays it was. One of the Chinese professors blamed the convenience foods as well as the foods imported from the West into Taiwan.

In a way, I was quite happy to hear this, as I had always felt that diet had so much bearing on this dreadful disease. When I told the lecturer about this particular incident, he responded by saying that China was a great distance away. I suggested we stay nearer home and look at the geographical distribution of Multiple Sclerosis and relate this to the intake of foods rich in linoleic acid or fatty acids, such as fish.

If we look at the Faroe Islands, we see that there is a very low incidence of Multiple Sclerosis. The Faroe Islanders have a Danish genetic background and remained fishermen. In our own Shetland Islands, however, a drastic change in diet took place, in line with agricultural influence from Britain. With the British diet, the Shetland Islanders acquired the British incidence of Multiple Sclerosis. Similarities are noticeable in the Netherlands and in Scandinavian countries.

Although Multiple Sclerosis occurs in most western countries, with a higher incidence in the cities, we cannot underestimate the fact that the highest percentage of Multiple Sclerosis is noted in the Orkneys and Shetlands in northern Scotland. In these particular areas, occurrence of Multiple Sclerosis is three times higher than in the rest of the UK, followed by New York City, which has the second highest rate in the world. It is also interesting to see that the intake of fat in the north of Scotland is 19 per cent greater than elsewhere in the United Kingdom and, of course, one cannot forget the fact that the intake of alcoholic drinks is very high in Scotland.

It is a fact that incidence of Multiple Sclerosis is low in tropical countries. This would appear not to relate so much to the temperature as to dietary management.

In 1960, a lady consulted us in our clinic in the Netherlands. She had made a remarkable recovery on a diet designed by Dr Evers from Germany. When I examined the diet regime, I noticed that the advised fat intake was very low. Large amounts of fresh fruit, fresh vegetables and grains were recommended. From that time on, we treated Multiple Sclerosis according to the Dr Evers methods and we achieved a certain measure of success.

After having settled in Britain over 30 years ago, a lady patient informed me that she had been following the Roger MacDougall diet. She followed his instructions carefully and had improved quite considerably. Of course, I was interested in her story and wrote to Roger MacDougall. He immediately replied with the message that he felt like a caller in the wilderness. After a lot of research and then strictly adhering to a gluten-free diet, he had achieved great success in his own management of the disease. Any assistance in establishing his diet and views would be most welcome.

I went to see him shortly after, on a visit to London, and could not believe my ears when I heard him running down the stairs. When he opened the front door, I found myself looking at a most active person and the thought immediately arose that if this man had spent a period of more than 20 years in a wheelchair, a miracle must have happened. After a long conversation with him, I came to the conclusion that this man did not just have a remission; the credit for his present condition must largely be ascribed to his dietary regime.

Later on, I had to go and see some Dutch patients who stayed in the Hilton Hotel and as we found we still had so much to discuss, he decided to come along with me. Both of us walked the length of Piccadilly and his step was faster than mine.

My curiosity about his methods was aroused and I decided to do some double tests. I put a group of people on the Evers diet and another group on the MacDougall diet. Undoubtedly, the last group made more progress than the first group and since that time, working along the lines of this dietary regime, some surprising successes have been achieved.

I do hope that from the following chapters Multiple Sclerosis sufferers will gain a little more enlightenment and will also learn the importance of eating the proper food. Several other methods which will help their condition are also described.

However, let there be no misunderstanding: Multiple Sclerosis is *not* curable. Let me quote Roger MacDougall on that point: 'As well try to cure a Chinaman of being Chinese. I was born a Sclerotic. It's in my genes. It's the hand I was dealt at conception with which to play out the game of life. Short of genetic engineering, I will die a Sclerotic. But I have lived a symptom-free life for quite a considerable number of years, except for a few brief lapses when I have been foolish enough and indulgent enough to break the rules. If I mistreat my body, it responds by renewing the old familiar symptoms – weirdly in exactly the reverse order in which they vanished. First to return is a touch of nystagmus (the last to go), then comes a slight paralysis in my right hand – my worst hand when I was crippled and the second last symptom to clear up. I've never dared to go on misbehaving and find out what would happen next.'

The important point then is that Multiple Sclerosis, though not curable by present drug-dependent medical methods, *is controllable*.

Preface to the 2002 edition

Today we live in the twenty-first century with a host of twenty-first century diseases. It is almost 35 years ago that I met Professor Roger MacDougall who performed a miracle because of his own logical thinking. His logic got him out of his wheelchair, when he was blind and crippled. With his own strict dietary management and the several things that he introduced, he lived to a ripe old age, very fit and very energetic. I have the greatest respect for this man, who did so much for others, especially when I receive letters daily, letters from people with this incurable disease, who have experienced relief or have made their condition controllable. Today there is still no cure for MS, yet the controllable improvements I see with MS patients are encouraging, showing how much diet can be of influence. Every day we read of more evidence on how the food we eat can influence our health pattern. When we look at how Roger warned us about the overuse of gluten and we look at several other health problems today – how right he was! It is an encouragement for everyone to go on and do one's best, to help oneself to better health.

Jan de Vries
June 2002

Prologue

Playwright, film writer, composer, lyricist, musician and Professor of Theatre Arts, Roger MacDougall was born in Bearsden, Dunbartonshire in 1910. His father, a headmaster in Glasgow, and his mother, a teacher, had hoped that their son would make a career in administrative education in Scotland. However, after studying at Glasgow University and graduating in law, he turned to writing and composing as a career and soon had numerous successes to his credit. He wrote plays, revues and sketches for the BBC, and music and lyrics for five revues at the Prince of Wales Theatre and two Crazy Gang Shows at the London Palladium.

It was inevitable that his talents would be snapped up by the busy British film studios. His pen was prolific and over the next few years he had no less than 26 screen credits to his name including *Midnight Menace*, *This Man is News* and *This Man in Paris*. At the famous Ealing Studios, he wrote several films, one of which was to become a screen classic, *The Man in the White Suit*, which starred Alec Guinness and for which Roger MacDougall received an Academy Award nomination. Other films followed including *The Gentle Gunman* (starring Dirk Bogard and Sir John Mills), *The Mouse that Roared* (starring Peter Sellers) and *A Touch of Larceny* (starring James Mason and George Sanders).

Constant demands from film studios did not mean that MacDougall neglected his first love, the theatre. His play, *To Dorothy, A Son* (later filmed with Shelley Winters), was a smash hit. It ran for 18 months, as did *Escapade* (which was later filmed with Sir John Mills and Alistair Sim).

It was just after *Escapade* had opened (in 1953) that Roger MacDougall was admitted to hospital for diagnosis of a strange deterioration in his eyesight and ability to walk properly. Multiple Sclerosis was diagnosed but the truth was kept from him. Only his wife, Renée, was told of his condition, while he was told he had 'inflammation of the nerves'. Slowly his condition worsened until he was a helpless invalid confined to a wheelchair. Defiant of his condition, he continued to work as best he could, dictating and using a tape recorder. By these means he wrote *The Facts of Life* and *A Touch of Larceny*.

Not content to accept the steady deterioration in his condition without question, it was inevitable that before long he learnt the truth – that he had Multiple Sclerosis. Refusing to believe that his condition was hopeless, MacDougall set out to evaluate his condition. At university, he had not studied medicine but he had studied logic, so that was the discipline he used, and this was his analysis. Because of his training, from anatomy onwards, a doctor naturally regards his patient as a sort of living cadaver with some flaw which is his job to correct. It might perhaps be more fruitful if he thought to consider that patient as a biochemical process going wrong, so that his job was to analyse and correct the biochemical process involved. Pursuing this biochemical approach, MacDougall went all the way back to the diet of the hunter-gatherer, the natural sustenance of our early ancestors, the diet from which modern man had progressed. As closely as he could, he reverted to it, and the effect he first noticed was that he stopped deteriorating. Encouraged, he continued it (primitive man did not have access to cows' milk or the various cereals which became available only after the agricultural revolution). So these and many other things like artificially treated foodstuffs had to be eliminated from his diet.

Four years passed and he got no worse. And then, still strictly following his diet, he began to improve. One day he managed to button the right-hand sleeve of his shirt. That was a memorable moment. The fingers of his left hand were coming to life! Then he found that he could stand erect without support. Next he could lift a pencil with his right hand. Soon he could actually write. And all the time his spectacles were becoming too strong, so he was forced to revert to lenses prescribed previously, when his eyesight was less affected. One by one his deadened faculties came back to life and, after a few more years, he was, as far as could be seen, back to normal.

Up to his death in May 1993, MacDougall remained in good health and as active as any normal man of his age. Was his return to normality an inexplicable remission as his neurologists would have him believe? Or was it as he maintained, the logical result of the diet he devised on his overworked auto-immune system – a defence overwhelmed by the allergens it had had to attack and destroy? This supposition is analogous to Professor Linus Pauling's theory of Orthomolecular Medicine.

Whatever the case, his approach to MS seems to have helped him in a really spectacular way. He remained positive, still walking about, still working, still reading and writing. It was only natural that he should hope that others will follow in his footsteps.

This is the story of Roger MacDougall's fight against Multiple Sclerosis and is in his own words.

'What follows is based upon my own experiences and the conclusion I drew from them. It should be clearly understood that I am not a doctor and have no medical training. My theories are controversial and, at this time, are not accepted by the medical profession. I obviously come in for much criticism from that quarter, which naturally distresses and depresses me. My aims were very simple – I suffered as all Multiple Sclerosis victims suffer and would therefore be inhuman if I did not try to offer whatever experience and advice I could to those still suffering.

'Some people question whether I ever actually had Multiple Sclerosis. Those of you who have Multiple Sclerosis and are suffering or have suffered the discomfort and indignities that result will identify and sympathise with the anger I feel at such a question. However, let me report the facts.

'I was diagnosed by Sir Charles Symonds at the National Hospital for Nervous Diseases in Queen Square, London, in February 1953. At that time, Sir Charles was recognised as one of the world's leading neurologists and Queen Square as one of the most celebrated neurological centres. Within a few years I was unable to use my legs, eyes and fingers – even my voice was affected – and I was quite unable to stand erect, even for a few seconds. Many years later, when I was living in Hollywood, I was given a thorough neurological examination – encephalograph, radioactive brain scanning, and lumbar puncture. Evidence of scar tissue damage was found in the brain and a sample of my spinal fluid was sent for analysis to a New York laboratory. It came back marked as a specimen from someone suffering from MS. What further proof can be required that I am in fact a victim of MS?

'Eight years after being pronounced terminal, my eyesight was restored, I could run up and down stairs and could lead as active a life as any man of my age. In support of these statements, I will refer later in this book to a medical examination I was given in September 1975 by a leading neurologist. No miracle has been performed. I have not been cured. I am simply experiencing a remission – but a remission which I firmly believe to be self-induced.

'While accepting that each person's body has a different metabolism, I feel it is not unreasonable to assume that the benefit I obtained, by following certain principles, may be applicable to others. (This may be borne out by the many people who write to tell me of their improvement.) I would be totally dishonest, however, if I claimed that the regime I describe in this book helps everyone who follows it. It appears to have helped me and many others. It is equally true to say that some people who have followed my recommendations have not in fact improved. To the best of my knowledge, they are a small minority and I am, of course, unsure that they followed my recommendations to the letter or for a sufficient length of time. My concern in those cases is paramount. However, since it took four years before I saw any real improvement in my own body, perhaps I may be forgiven for wondering whether others had the same determination to succeed as I had. It is true to say that with those who write to tell me of their improvements, progress is often discouragingly slow. However, a slow improvement is clearly to be preferred to a slow deterioration.

'It must be said that many people who do not follow my regime, who may indeed never have heard about it, experience spontaneous remissions of varying duration. The doctors cannot explain these remissions and I would not presume to attempt to. This does not, however, in any way shake my belief that the approach to my own condition described in this book was largely responsible for the spectacular improvement I have experienced.'

WHAT IS THIS CONDITION MULTIPLE SCLEROSIS?

'There appears to be no generally accepted understanding of the cause. It has to be defined by describing its effects. According to *Black's Medical Dictionary*: "It consists of hardened patches, from the size of a pinhead to that of a pea or larger, scattered here and there irregularly through the brain and (spinal) cord, each patch being made up of a mass of the connective tissue (neuroglia), which should be present only in sufficient amount to bind the nerve cells and fibres together. In the earliest stage, the insulating sheaths of the nerve fibres in the hardened patches break up, are absorbed, and leave the nerve fibres bare, the connective tissue being later formed between these. The actual changes in the nervous system appear to be due to the action of some substance which dissolves or breaks up the fatty matter of the nerve sheaths." Or according to *Gould's* (Blakestons's 3rd Edition): "Demyelinisation followed by gliosis and formation of plaques affecting different parts of the nervous system in patches. Cause unknown."

'In simple terms, it would appear that the insulation of the nerve deteriorates so that the impulses can no longer be effectively carried to and from the brain. The result may be paralysis, partial blindness, lack of balance and the whole familiar range of symptoms which can vary widely from case to case. Let there be no misunderstanding, Multiple Sclerosis is incurable, about this there can be no question. I, however, could not accept what appeared to be the inevitability of spending the rest of my life slowly deteriorating in a wheelchair. I knew I could not cure my condition, so what I tried to do was control it. This I appear to have done.

'What was the thinking behind my approach and how did I set about it? As earlier stated, I have had no medical training. I was, however, trained in logic, after taking my law degree at Glasgow University, and this training was of considerable help to me in developing my approach. Logic told me that, since Multiple Sclerosis was apparently caused by the breakdown of the myelin sheath surrounding the nerves, it was likely to be a degenerative condition. I also suspected that Multiple Sclerosis was as much a biochemical problem as a medical one. More specifically, I assumed that Multiple Sclerosis was caused by a chemical imbalance resulting in the inability of the body to create replacement tissue for the myelin layer surrounding the nerves. In other words, I came to regard the body as a chemical process and Multiple Sclerosis as a manifestation of that chemical process going wrong.

'These suppositions led me to believe that Multiple Sclerosis might be controlled by adjusting the food intake in a way which would correct the offending chemical imbalance. I therefore decided that I should pursue those approaches, which were not only medically acceptable in the treatment of other degenerative conditions, but were also compatible with my hunter-gatherer concept. These were:

A gluten-free diet, which removes the symptoms of coeliac disease.
A sugar-free diet, which is indicated in cases of diabetes and hypoglycaemia.
A diet free of milk fat which appears to help those with cardiovascular conditions.

'The resultant approach was based on two objectives. Firstly, to remove from the diet ingredients which I believe to be harmful – gluten, dairy products and refined sugar. Secondly, to eat good natural foodstuffs which would replace nutrients that might otherwise be lost as a result of following the diet. It should be remembered that in cutting out foods that contain what I believe to be harmful ingredients, one may at the same time deprive oneself of otherwise valuable foodstuffs. I will elaborate on this point later.

'Over the course of the next few years, I dropped the suspect foods from my diet one after another. At first I merely stabilised the state of my symptoms; then, slowly and steadily, my health improved. Slowly is the word I must emphasise. It was more than four years before I noticed the first significant improvement, when I managed to fumble a shirt-sleeve button into the buttonhole – the first time my fingers had obeyed a command for a very long time. Thus encouraged, I took a closer interest in the problem of nutrition in relation to my condition.

'Over the years, I refined my dietary recommendations in the light of my own experiences and other people's, and the dos and don'ts which follow are those which I believe offer the best chance of improvement to the broadest spectrum of Multiple Sclerosis sufferers. I owe a great deal – everything in fact – to the work of many different doctors, biochemists, scientists, research workers and nutritional experts. I have merely put together into a cohesive pattern discoveries, suggestions and realisations which have come from many others. It is a positive approach to the problem and one which appears to be helping large numbers of people. By its very nature, it is often extremely slow in showing results but, as I have said earlier, a slow improvement is surely preferable to a slow, hopeless degeneration. I hope that one day soon the medical profession will test my theories by practical methods which will take into account biochemical and dietetic considerations.

'I have followed the course dictated by my theories for many years and, in evidence of my present state of health, I am delighted to tell you that in September 1975 I went to the neurologist who, in 1953, was Sir Charles Symond's assistant and actually conducted most of my original examination at Queen Square. I asked him to give me a complete and thorough neurological examination. This he did, and throughout the examination kept saying "I can't fault you". Every reflex, every muscle, every movement was normal. Finally, he came to my eyes and at the extremity of my field of vision, as I glanced right, he found a vestigial trace of nystagmus (juddering of the optic nerve). When, at my worst, I had suffered from nystagmus to the point of virtual blindness, so that to be left with a vestigial trace, of which I am totally unaware, hardly presents a hardship. As far as my eyes are otherwise concerned, my astigmatism has cleared up amazingly and I am now able, in good sunlight, to read newsprint without glasses – something I have not been able to do for more than 30 years. At the conclusion of my examination, the neurologist confirmed that this slight trace of nystagmus was the only damage that appeared to remain throughout my entire system as the result of a crippling attack of Multiple Sclerosis. Talking about the past, he recalled that I'd had a pretty severe episode in the years that followed our first meeting at Queen Square. I asked him point-blank if he'd ever encountered such a spectacular remission and he freely admitted that he hadn't.

'What am I suggesting then to victims of Multiple Sclerosis? Certainly not the possibility of a cure – though that should not be far away. Experiments in "genetic engineering" seem certain to find a faulty gene which can be corrected. Meanwhile, I at least offer the possibility of a complete reversal and 100 per cent control of the symptoms – not too much different from a cure, as I have found. At first, I thought I had indeed cured myself, but a few days back indulging my former eating habits and the paralysis began to return to my right hand – the last symptom to clear away. This was clear enough warning, and since then I have stuck rigidly to my diet.'

DIET

'It is important that I should point out here that, through no wish of my own, I have become known to many people as "the gluten-free man", with the implication that the banning of gluten is the be-all and end-all of my approach to Multiple Sclerosis. Nothing could be further from the truth. A gluten-free diet on its own could in fact be extremely harmful, leading, among other things, to a serious loss of B vitamins in which Sclerotics are already deficient, and to a serious loss of weight. You must remember that the removal of gluten from your diet – although in my view essential – is only one aspect of the complete approach. I believe that the dietary approach to degenerative conditions should take the form of a four-pronged attack:

1. No gluten.
2. Low sugars.
3. Low animal fats. High unsaturated fats.
4. Compensating for possible vitamin/mineral deficiencies.

'It is medically accepted that certain conditions are caused or aggravated by the consumption of certain foods. For example, coeliac disease linked with cereals, diabetes and hypoglycaemia linked with sugar, cardiovascular conditions linked with dairy fats. My regime is based on the belief that Multiple Sclerosis falls into the same category but, again, it must be stressed that this opinion is not shared by medical authority. If I am right, it is surely possible that you are eating foods to which you may be allergic and which may be doing you harm. I believe that, by eating the correct foods, you will have a good chance of improving your condition. As with so much in life, success must depend on your own determination and there can be no half-hearted approximation to the rules. Watch every dish you eat lest it contains one of the substances I believe to be harmful. If you are tempted to cheat, remember you are only cheating yourself. Once you have corrected your diet, you will find it almost as easy to follow as your present one. That too is only a matter of habit. Good or bad eating habits – the choice is yours.'

SUPPLEMENTARY VITAMINS AND MINERALS

'As I have said earlier, it is important that anyone following the diet should not, by cutting out the undesirable foods I mention later, cut out also any of the beneficial vitamins and minerals those foods contain along with their harmful ingredients. For example, milk – which I believe to be harmful because of its animal fat content – is, at the same time, a valuable source of Vitamin B2, B12 and Calcium. The ideal way to counter the problem is, of course, to eat other foods which contain the necessary vitamins and minerals, but which are not in any way harmful due to the presence of deleterious ingredients. However, as I soon discovered, this is not always possible and, furthermore, one may find that some of these foods are unacceptable purely from the point of view of personal taste. (How many of us, for example, can stomach a daily ration of raw chopped liver?)

'It was to combat these difficulties that, with the assistance and guidance of a doctor friend, I set about formulating a simple tablet which would contain a broad spectrum of the vitamins and minerals most likely to be lost as a result of rigid adherence to my diet. I list below the ingredients that we settled upon, together with the amounts contained in each tablet. I do this for two reasons:

1. To show that there is no magical ingredient included
   – simply well-known vitamins and minerals.
2. To guide those who might feel that they would
   rather buy the ingredients themselves.

'I personally found it quite impracticable, and very costly, to buy all the ingredients separately and in the right proportions, not to mention the fact that it would have involved the consumption of a very large number of tablets each day. Here is the basic formula I devised:

Choline Bitartrate 10.0 mg Vitamin B1 2.0 mg Vitamin B2 1.0 mg Vitamin B6 6.0 mg Vitamin B12 0.015 mg Vitamin C 25.0 mg Vitamin E 7.5 mg Inositol 10.0 mg Folic Acid 0.04 mg Nicotinamide 40.0 mg Calcium-D-Pantothenate 12.0 mg Calcium Gluconate 75.0 mg Magnesium Carbonate 75.0 mg Lecithin 25.0 mg
(I take four of these tablets three times daily).

'It has been brought to my attention that some people are under the impression the tablets which I formulated are sold as a cure for Multiple Sclerosis. This has never been the case. Let me make it quite clear once and for all – the tablets I suggest are designed and intended solely to supplement the intake of vitamins and minerals in which some people may find themselves deficient as a result of strict adherence to the diet I recommend.

'Having said this, I must make the point that it is generally accepted in medical circles that Sclerotics are deficient in certain vitamins, especially the B group, and I would be doing you a disservice if I did not point out that following my diet to the letter could further deplete your intake of these vitamins.

'I am concerned that you should replace these possible losses. Whether you eat more good natural foods, buy your own vitamins and minerals or buy the tablets that I use is unimportant. What is important is that you should not underestimate or neglect the importance of this aspect of a balanced diet.'

WHAT TO AVOID
'In this section, I deal specifically with foods I cut out from my own diet because I believed they were doing me harm, i.e. those that contain either gluten, high animal fats or refined sugar. The list looks formidable and will almost certainly involve fundamental changes in your present eating habits, but you will see from the following section headed 'What You Can Eat' that

the range of good, nourishing and tasty foods still available to you is very wide and permits plenty of variation in your daily menus.

'You must cut out gluten rigidly. That means you should avoid all use of *wheat*, *barley*, *oats* and *rye*, all of which contain gluten, and this includes foods made from or containing these grains or the gluten from them, such as Weetabix, Shredded Wheat, Wheat Germ Flakes, Froment, All-Bran, white and brown bread, cakes, puddings, biscuits, porridge, rye and wheat crispbreads, all kinds of pasta, semolina, Bisto, etc. Eat nothing that has even a pinch of flour in it. In this respect your diet must be as strict as that of someone suffering from coeliac disease.

'Completely cut out all refined sugar – white or demerara – and all foods containing it, such as jams, marmalades, cakes, biscuits, tinned fruit, sweets, chocolate, ice-cream, glacé cherries and candied fruits. Try to restrict yourself to very small amounts of unrefined sugar – soft brown, Barbados, Turbinado, Muscovado, etc. – honey, or pure maple syrup.

'You should severely limit your intake of all animal fats. Cut out butter, cream and rich cheeses. Fresh milk should not be taken because it contains too much fat or cream, so use only skimmed milk, skimmed milk powder or goats' milk. Instead of butter, use margarine made from sunflower seed, safflower seed oil for cooking and salads. Use any vegetable oil, preferably sunflower oil. Fried foods are the hardest to digest, so please try to reduce your intake.

'Bacon too should be avoided. Whenever you desire, you can eat free range animals (venison, rabbit, poultry) in preference to farmed animals. Always remember to remove the fat from your meat and don't take pork, duck or goose.

'In farmed animals, the ratio of adipose (harmful) fat to structural (essential) fat can be 50 to one. In free range animals it is two to one.

'Beer, gin, whisky, vodka, sweetened fruit juices and bottled fizzy drinks are not permitted.'

WHAT YOU CAN EAT

'Gluten-free cereals, such as rice, maize and millet and products made from these cereals – such as rice flour, cornflour, maize flour, etc. are all permissible.

'Brown natural rice can be used as a basic cereal food. It contains 9½ times more minerals than polished refined white rice. You can eat such breakfast foods as Corn Flakes, Rice Krispies, Puffed Rice or Millet Flakes. These do, however, contain a minimal amount of sugar, so it would be wise not to eat too much of them.

'Many health stores, especially in America, sell very palatable gluten-free bread made from rice flour, maize flour, soya bean flour, millet flour, potato flour and lima bean flour – or some combination of these. They are all permissible and can all be home-baked.

'You can eat all *vegetables*, fresh and frozen, including potatoes, which are best cooked in their skins. Try not to overcook vegetables. They are best steamed in only a little water, and eaten when still crisp. (Canned vegetables are usually less nutritious and often contain additives.) If you make fries (chips), they should be cooked in fresh vegetable oil – such as sunflower or safflower seed oil. Potato crisps are probably made with saturated oil, so I suggest you use them with discretion.

'You can eat all salad foods in large quantities. These are a fine source of additional natural minerals and vitamins.

'You can eat all *fruits* – fresh, frozen and dried. To reconstitute evaporated (dehydrated) fruit: Wash fruit. Put in a heatproof dish with lid. Cover fruit with boiling water and replace lid. Leave for 24 to 48 hours when it is ready to serve. *Do not cook.* Fruit canned in honey is also acceptable. Always eat your apple pips – they are rich in linoleic acid. Linoleic also exists in other seeds and in the tips of growing things – like bean sprouts. Linoleic acid is found in dark green leafy vegetables.

'What you need are the long-chain polyunsaturated lipids – linoleic, linolenic and arachidonic acids – the so-called fatty acids.

'You can also drink *fruit and vegetables juices* so long as they do not contain added sugar. Some good ones are apple juice, grape juice, carrot juice and beetroot juice.

'Comb honey is better than clear honey. In order to facilitate bottling and to increase shelf life, manufacturers heat clear honey to 180°. This effectively destroys many of its nutrients, and yet it can still legally be sold as 'raw honey'. This is why I try to avoid many other processed foods. In order to increase shelf life their food value is often drastically reduced.

'You can eat lean beef, lamb, liver, kidneys, etc., chicken and fish, eggs and egg dishes. Try not to eat too much beef though, as it contains acids which are not helpful to good health. Canned meat (corned beef or tongue) is perfectly all right. Liver paté is permissible if it does not contain monosodium glutamate.

'All fresh *fish* is permitted. Canned fish (sardines, kippers, salmon, tuna, etc.) is allowed, though not ideal. (I hope that some day fish may be available canned in vegetable oil.)

'Sago and tapioca are permitted.

'Wheatgerm oil is allowed, but not wheatgerm flakes.

'You can eat cottage cheese and yoghurt, but not too much ordinary cheese because of the fat content – and please avoid rich creamy cheeses (Brie, Camembert, Port Salut, etc.).

'Nuts – except Brazil and cashew nuts which are high in saturated fats – are excellent for protein, minerals and vitamins.

'Chocolate made from raw sugar may be taken, though not too much of it. Candy made from carob is preferable. Sunflower seeds and pumpkin seeds are excellent "nibblers" as substitutes for sweets.

'Artificial sweeteners are not better or worse for Multiple Sclerosis patients than they are for anyone else. This covers drinks, dietetic foods, etc. The decision to take them or leave them alone is entirely yours.

'Tea and coffee can be taken, but decaffeinated coffee is preferable. Use buttermilk. This is an alkali-forming food which contains sodium and lecithin and combats acidosis. Marmite or other yeast extracts may be used as a drink. Permissible alcoholic drinks include cider, sherry, wine, brandy, Campari, Cinzano, Dubonnet and other vermouths.

'*Always read the labels before purchasing any processed food.* Natural food is always to be preferred. If you have to eat processed food, make sure it does not contain any forbidden ingredient. This would apply especially to mayonnaise, ketchups, catsups, sauces, etc.'

WEIGHT

'It is vitally important that you watch your weight. Although most people following the diet remain approximately the same weight, some actually gain weight – others lose it. The following observations are addressed to those who may lose weight until they are beneath the normal weight for their height.

'Stay off dairy products, but relax the ban on animal fat.

'Eat as many of the legumes as possible – haricot beans, butter beans, the old stand-by Heinz beans, and any others. Also eat lentils, both yellow and brown, and chick-peas. Don't forget that natural rice is a valuable body-building food.

'Take tapioca and sago, made with reconstituted skimmed milk and Barbados sugar.

'Eat plenty of potatoes, preferably baked or steamed in their skins.

'Tinned soya beans, soya bean flour for thickening soups and gravies, and soya bean oil are nourishing foods.

'And Popeye wasn't wrong – spinach helps build muscles too.

'Still eat meat from wild animals, like venison, rabbit or hare, and free-range poultry, in preference to domestic meats.

'And still eat offal – liver, kidneys, tripe, brains, etc. – in preference to meats like pork and veal and even steak and lamb.

'However, any dietician should be able to advise you on how to remain at your correct weight without going against the diet. If you develop a weight problem, it is best to get professional advice.'

GENERAL HEALTH HINTS

'Whenever possible, eat foods as fresh as possible. Eat raw

vegetables, such as shredded cabbage, raw grated carrots and beetroot. Eat fresh fruits every day too – they give you live enzymes which aid digestion.

'Fruit and vegetable juices are a fine "liquid meal". Fresh juices can be extracted from vegetables with a juice extractor or you can purchase them in a health food shop. Natural (unsweetened) juices are sugar free and can give an additional daily intake of Vitamin C.

'Frequent baths with suitable additives such as sea salt, sauna baths and physiotherapy are helpful in stimulating circulation and eliminating waste matter from the body.

'Fresh air is a gift from Nature. If you are able, get out into the country. Trees take in carbon dioxide, a waste from our bodies, and give off fresh oxygen, so it must do you good to be amongst them.

'Remember, your degenerative condition has taken many years to show itself, so you won't improve overnight.

'You will need patience, perseverance and diligent application of yourself to the diet. If you cheat, you are cheating no one but yourself. I follow the diet to this day, and nothing on earth would make me give it up. It helped me; it seems to be helping many others. I hope it will help you.'

SECOND THOUGHTS

'It may seem odd to start at the end of a complex story, the story of my life, but perhaps that is the only place to start if I am to convey the truth.

'Here I am, aged 82, anxious to outline the potential explanations of the tragic incidents which struck me down at the very moment when my career as a playwright seemed set fair. I was just enjoying my first long-running hit – *To Dorothy, A Son* – which was to stay a success at the Garrick Theatre for more than 18 months.

'It was then, 40 years ago, that my life changed irrevocably. I was unable to stand erect even for a second. I had difficulty in enunciating words, my eyesight was plagued with nystagmus so that I could not recognise faces more than a foot away. My hands and arms were almost completely paralysed, I was not even capable of holding a pencil, let alone write, and the sum total of symptoms suggested that I had suffered a stroke, but my condition was diagnosed as the final stages of a virulent attack of inflammation of the nerves.

'The orthodox treatment prescribed for me and which, for a time, I endured, was as follows:

'Firstly, I was given intramuscular injections of Vitamin B12. Then I received a transfusion of fresh, living blood transferred directly from the donor to me. After that a colourless liquid was administered four times a day. This had disastrous effects on my digestive system. I felt constantly sick and unwell. I suffered this for some time before asking my neurologist what it was I was being given. "Arsenic," he replied without batting an eyelid. Then, seeing my startled reaction, by way of justification he added: "It's a well-known treatment for nervous problems."

'I had a vague memory of having read somewhere that once arsenic is consumed it remains in the body permanently. Whether this is true or not I have no idea, but at that particular moment his reply did nothing to reassure me. As can readily be imagined, I grew less and less enchanted with the neurological approach, but in a hospital situation the layman feels hopeless.

'Then one day, when my wife visited me, she burst into tears and confessed that I had not been told the truth: I was suffering from Multiple Sclerosis and the prognosis was simply continuous deterioration. My reaction to this was to become furious with the medics for what I looked upon as their unforgivable arrogance in concealing my true condition from me.

'What were they implying? That only they could do anything for me? And what had they done so far? Nothing at all. I had simply been used as a guinea pig. Then I asked my wife to collect my goods and chattels and take me home.

'At age 15, I had passed my University Entrance Examination and, with three other boys from my class, came up to Glasgow University. Probably because of the influence of my mother and father (he had been headmaster of a Glasgow school and my mother had been a teacher), I had always come first in exams. Once at university, I started on an ambitious programme my father had worked out for me. He had taken a simple MA degree and felt that his lack of qualifications had held him back in his career, so he planned that I should try for an Honours Degree in English, together with degrees in Law and Education.

'When I completed studying for my ambitious courses, I began to sit for my finals. Unfortunately, my eyesight failed and I experienced double vision. Though I did not realise it at the time, this was the first outbreak of my latent Multiple Sclerosis. The condition of my eyes cleared up temporarily, but I decided not to return to university. I had had the education, I told myself, and that was more important than the degrees.

'Had I remained under the influence of the Queen Square neurologists, I would never have devised the therapy which appears to have strengthened my immune system to the point where it banished the symptoms of MS from me (as, subsequently, it has for many others). In addition, the same regime also alleviates and, indeed, can remove the symptoms of many other degenerative conditions.

'How did I arrive at my "therapy"? Going back to my school pal, now a doctor, as soon as he had the chance, he took me into the anatomy lab at Glasgow University in an attempt to shock me by showing me a cadaver. Years later this incident crossed my mind as I was thinking about my predicament. I realised that my doctors were conditioned to look upon me as a cadaver suffering from a disease of the nervous system, whereas I looked upon myself as a biochemical process which had gone wrong. This led me to the conclusion that I should not be searching for a drug to attack the "disease", but for the correct nutrients to restore my chemical balance. After further thought, I also concluded that I was not an Upper Primate – eating the natural food of such a species, but was instead eating what pleased me solely by its taste.

'I thereupon set about making the necessary revolutionary

changes in my diet. I cut out all ingredients which had proved harmful in other contexts – like gluten in coeliac disease, sugar in diabetes, milk fat in heart conditions. Finally I added a number of vitamins and minerals, mainly to restore essentials I had removed, such as calcium and the B vitamins. For some years all that happened was that the deterioration in my condition did not worsen. I had stopped degenerating as had been predicted. There was no marked improvement, but I am an obstinate-minded Scotsman and I stuck it out, remaining convinced that this was the logical course to continue.

'After four or five years of perseverance, my reward began to show itself. My symptoms began to vanish "like snow in summer" as a clergyman who followed my method tellingly expressed it.

'Before too long, I regained my old faculties. I was able to bound up the stairs, play tennis again, and behave like any normal, healthy man of 50. Another benefit I experienced from therapy, if I may so call it, was that it slowed down the ageing process. After a routine examination by my optician, to his surprise he found that the glasses he had previously prescribed were now too strong for me. My skin, which had begun to wrinkle and age, became soft and youthful again, and I need hardly add that I was once again able to walk normally. But let me immediately emphasise that I am not claiming, and never have claimed, to be able to "cure" Multiple Sclerosis, only to control and reverse the process.

'Friends I happened to help by their following my own example encouraged me to set up a small company called Regenics. I wrote my first booklet and began to manufacture a multi-mineral and vitamin tablet, which led to a postal service for fellow victims. Because I was a successful playwright, the story of my recovery received publicity and the account was eventually picked up by the *National Enquirer* in the United States. Copies of my booklet had already been sent to MS victims over there in response to letters I had received. The booklet itself was a factual account of my experiences and made no claims whatsoever.

'It remains my conviction that unless some so far unidentified virus (perhaps too minute even for the electron microscope to reveal) is found to be responsible, Multiple Sclerosis will only be "cured" when genetic research discovers some damaged gene which can be corrected or replaced. I am aware that Parkinson's Disease has been found to be caused by a gene which can be restored by the introduction of foetal material and perhaps, one day, some equally good answer may be produced for Multiple Sclerosis. In my mind, there is no doubt whatsoever that MS is not a disease of the nerves. It is a disease which ends up in the nerves but which starts off with the failure of the body to build the correct replacement tissue for the myelin sheaths which insulate the nerves. Calling in a neurologist to deal with such a condition is like asking an electrician to deal with a plumbing defect, or consulting a dermatologist to deal with scarlet fever because of the strange colour of the skin!

'Therefore my most important piece of thinking was to realise that MS is not a Cause, but a Result – the result of my failure to supply my digestive system with the ingredients I needed in order to build new cell tissue, which in turn would maintain the myelin sheaths around my nerves. I have never been able to accept the official medical opinion that MS is subject to inexplicable "remissions". This simply means, it seems to me, that so far doctors have been unable to understand or explain why MS is subject to such variations.

'You may ask how I devised my own regime.

'Aspects of the "You are what you eat" school began to occupy my thoughts. A tiger eats nothing but meat. Feed it on grass and it will die. Similarly, if you were to feed a cow on meat, the cow would die, since its digestive system can only assimilate grass. When I saw the first pathetic shots of a cow with the so-called "Mad Cow Disease" on television, I said "There goes a silly cow called Roger MacDougall," and meant it. We were told by experts that the cow's condition was caused by the introduction of animal waste into its feed, and that somehow it had acquired "scrapie" from infected foodstuffs. Obviously, utter nonsense! It had been fed on a diet it was not designed by nature to cope with, just like the tiger fed on grass, or me feeding myself with my particular allergens – milk fat and gluten. Poor cow, I thought, just like poor me before I took myself in hand and stopped relying on the experts' opinions.

'Over the long years, I have frequently wondered why it was left to me, a layman, to find a way of easing my own misery and in fact saving my own life? In my initial euphoria at having drastically improved my pitiful condition, I believed I had found a way of dealing with MS, but I later realised that the same method could materially help other degenerative states as well. It suddenly dawned on me that my self-experiments had found a way of dealing with the auto-immune system.

'What it comes down to is this: over the past 35 years I have effectively controlled the effects of MS through diet. Why do I say "controlled" rather than "cured"? Very simply, because whenever I reverted to my previous diet, the symptoms returned, but if I faithfully stuck to my strict rules I continued to regain normality. If I relaxed and ate bread and milk fat products, the progress was halted. It may be difficult for people to believe I found the strength of purpose to act on such initial, slight encouragement, but I did and I am still here to tell the tale.

'In so far as my opinion has value, it seems clear to me that we allow a rather loose use of the word "disease". It would seem more reasonable to define complaints more rationally. Thus, where the cause is the invasion of a germ or virus, the word "infection" might be appropriate, whereas a condition caused autonomously by the breakdown of the person's own system without any outside influence might then, more reasonably, be called a "disease".

'In time, conditions brought about by faulty diet could be differentiated. This opens up an intriguing field in which the mystery some doctors tend to encourage would necessarily vanish. What is scurvy, for instance? And when it comes down to it, what is cancer and what is AIDS? – diseases or infections, or what? It would force the medical world to think more specifically.

'MS, as I see it, is the effect of an inborn condition. As well to try and cure a Chinaman of being Chinese as to try and cure an MS victim of being a Multiple Sclerotic. A Chinaman is what he is, just as a Sclerotic is what I am. I am a person whose myelin sheaths harden and deteriorate, unless I follow a strict intake of nutrients. I don't think I can put it more clearly than that.

'I have to keep underlining that I am writing about the "care" and not the "cure" of someone who was diagnosed as an MS victim. But the care I can offer results in freedom from symptoms and that, in turn, makes it clear, to me at any rate, that neurologists are simply wasting time and money unless they research the genetic approach to a complete answer, and the same is sadly true of the good people who run the Multiple Sclerosis Society. What patients should be told in the first instance is that they have *had* MS and are now suffering from its effects. The logical course is not to attack MS but what *caused* it – and what caused it was the failure of the individual's metabolism to provide him or her with replacement cell tissue for the insulation of the nerves: i.e. the myelin which the sclerosis hardened and made ineffectual.

'It is my small but fervent hope that once professional minds stop fighting the truth of my attitude, they will set about improving on the amateurish stumbling which led to my recovery. I don't even claim that my way is necessarily the best way, only that it is the way I found which cleared my symptoms completely and which, subsequently, has helped hundreds of others. I can cause the symptoms to happen to my body at will; I can cause the symptoms to vanish from my body in a few weeks if I do not allow them to get too far; I can cause them to vanish from the bodies of others if they have only recently appeared. Those who care to adopt my therapy can expect a happy outcome: their symptoms will first stop regressing and then, if they persevere, will begin to disappear.

'I am now in my eighty-second year and I am still keeping my symptoms at bay, so I feel I am entitled to claim victory which enabled me to continue a productive and creative life for 40 years beyond what I had been told was my allotted span. We are often told we should be grateful for small mercies. Well, in my case, the mercy was anything but small, and I would like to think that my unaided experiments will have a life beyond my own and bring some measure of comfort and help to others. If so, then I shall depart knowing that my efforts have not been in vain.

'I had the enormous advantage of training in logic instead of in medicine. Consequently I did not accept the preconceived conclusions about my condition, but instead I worked things out from scratch. Also I had my own damaged body to observe on a day-to-day basis and could study the effects of whatever actions I took.

'Despite the fact that an increasing number of doctors now accept that the intake of nutrients plays a vital role in combating many of the ailments that flesh is heir to, there are still those who refuse to admit that there is something beyond the orthodox approach. Why should this continue to be? I think the answer is many of them expect diet to conform to the so-called "scientific approach" – the randomised double-blind trial with placebo substitution – conveniently ignoring the fact that the human metabolism is much too complicated for that to be a viable route. What helps "A" may not help "B". Even more complicated is the possibility that a certain substance may help "B" only if it is introduced in complement with something else and may have no beneficial effect unless the other substance is also present.

'This principle of "team work" in diet is examined at length by Roger J. Williams, James D. Heffley, Man Li Yew and Charles W. Bode in a paper headed *Perspectives in Biology and Medicine. A Renaissance of Nutritional Science is Imminent.*

'I owe the confirmation of the validity of my own thinking to their work, and I am sure they would be only too happy for me to quote from their observations.

> There is a wide spectrum of uninformed, inexpert opinion regarding the practical importance of quality nutrition in our daily lives. At one extreme are the food enthusiasts, including faddists; at the other is the

39

majority of practising physicians who, through the fault of their medical school training, tend to ignore all but the most elementary aspects of nutrition and to avoid becoming involved in a field so characterised by intricacies, uncertainties and ignorance.

'This, as I have already noted, confirmed conclusions I had already reached in my attempt to find a logical alternative to the original diagnosis of my condition. I could not accept the statement that MS is subject to "inexplicable remissions". In my view, we live in a causally connected universe and therefore all any doctor is entitled to say is that MS is subject to remission *for reasons he is so far unable to explain.*

'The Roger Williams paper goes on to say:

> Those who have medical training are in a unique position. They alone have the background necessary fully to grasp the deep-seated significance of nutrition in relation to health and disease. Unfortunately, however, medical science and the public has all too often discovered that those who should know the most about nutrition know very little.

'Later on comes this passage:

> An inspired writer in the *Heinz Handbook of Nutrition* wrote 36 years ago as follows:
> 'Individual organisms differ in their genetic make-up and differ also in morphologic and physiologic aspects, including their endocrine activity, metabolic efficiency and nutritional requirements. It is often taken for granted that the human population is made up of individuals who exhibit average physiologic requirements and that a minor proportion of the population is composed of those whose requirements may be considered to deviate excessively. Actually there is little justification in nutritional thinking for the

concept that a representative prototype of Homo sapiens is one who has average requirements with respect to all essential nutrients and thus exhibits no unusually high or low needs. In the light of contemporary genetic physiologic knowledge and the statistical interpretation thereof, the typical individual is more likely to be one who has average needs with respect to many essential nutrients, but who also exhibits some nutritional requirements for a few essential nutrients which are far from average.'

'Finally, I'd like to address myself, not to sufferers, but to those who can help them. The future seems set, and many neurologists are working towards a solution. My concern is with the present. Like Martin Luther King, I have a dream, a dream in which those neurologists not engaged in research will begin to help their patients towards resuming a normal life as I succeeded in doing. They are so much better qualified for the job than I was. I wonder how many of them have received as many heart-warming letters as I have from people they have helped.'

EPILOGUE
An extract from Bryan Forbes' latest autobiography, *A Divided Life*. It is his account of his recovery from Multiple Sclerosis after following the Roger MacDougall programme. We feel sure you will be encouraged by reading this chapter.

It was a perfect summer's day in July, the eve of my 49th birthday, when the specialist delivered the verdict that I had Multiple Sclerosis.

The first disturbing symptoms had occurred a month or so previously while I was shooting the snow sequences for *The Slipper and the Rose* high in the Austrian Alps near Anif. I became aware that something was odd when, returning by the hotel after work, I stepped into a hot bath which mysteriously felt ice cold. Conversely, when my bare flesh touched the rim of the porcelain washbasin, I felt a searing burn. It was as if wires had been crossed and I was receiving contra-reactions. A day or so later I developed agonising sensations in my right leg as though a fire was raging within. My eyes were also affected and I began to lose my balance.

Every film director is compelled to take a rigorous medical examination before shooting commences, and it is a contractual requirement that the insurance company be immediately notified of any subsequent conditions that might jeopardise the progress of the film. I forced myself to believe it was just a temporary aberration brought on by an intensive work schedule in bitter weather, and bent the rules by first consulting my own doctor on my return home. He sent me to a neurologist who proved to be a somewhat dingy individual with a marked lack of bedside manner. After he had prodded and stuck needles into me, he said gloomily, 'Well, one can't rule out cancer of the spine, or even the possibility of a brain tumour. You'll have to have some extensive tests and go on the scanner.'

After this horrifying prognosis, my condition deteriorated. I began actually to fall down, my eyesight weakened and I was compelled to notify the film insurance company, although I did not stop working. They demanded I had further tests, so every day before going to the studio I was seen by at least six specialists at various hospitals, none of whom came up with any conclusive diagnosis. Finally, they pooled all their findings and one of them was delegated to come to my home and pronounce sentence. There had been no further change in my condition; apart from pains in my right leg, I felt reasonably well and convinced myself I had picked up some rare bug which the medicos would eventually isolate and treat with modern drugs.

It was a Sunday evening in July, when the light has

special qualities, that the spokesman came to Seven Pines. Nanette was out when he arrived and he made a special point of saying he would wait for her to return before telling me the decision reached. I took this to mean good news. When Nanette eventually came back, he asked us both to sit together and then he began to read a typed statement, rather like a governor of a prison telling a condemned man that all appeals had been exhausted and the execution would now go forward. My first reaction was anger, not so much at the verdict but the manner in which it had been broken to me in front of Nanette.

'So what is the treatment?' I managed to say. At that point I was very ignorant about the disease.

'The first thing is you must give up work. It's important that you don't have any stress.'

'If I give up work, you won't be paid,' I heard myself saying, 'so I wouldn't suggest that. What else can be done?'

'The standard treatment is cortisone,' he replied.

Again I heard myself saying, 'I'm not taking that. I'm told it has disastrous side effects. What's the alternative?'

'At the moment, very little, although research is going on all the time.'

The rest of the conversation remains hazy, but I know that I dismissed him shortly afterwards and never consulted him again. Apparently, when showing him out, Nanette asked how long I had to live and he gave a bleak answer. Throughout the next two years, Nanette's anguish was far worse than mine because, from the moment I was told, I became bloody-minded and refused to believe the worst.

The following morning I was scheduled to shoot one of the large musical numbers in the presence of Her Majesty Queen Elizabeth, the Queen Mother, Princess Margaret and her two children, all of whom were paying a rare visit to the studio. I got through that day somehow and the curious thing is that while I was on the set and concentrating on the direction of the film, all the symptoms disappeared. It was only at the end of the day that they returned. This further strengthened my resolve to rely on mind over matter, a potent force for good.

The only person I told was my producer, Stuart Lyons, and he agreed to keep the confidence. I promised him, with God knows what justification, that I would finish the film come what may and he agreed to share the risk. I had no idea what came next or how long I could continue to function but trusted to luck and willpower.

Nanette refused to trust to luck and, although greatly distressed, she set to work to find the answer. Everything that followed I owe to her. I have to be careful how I set down the rest of the story because I am told that there could still be an element of risk to the main character involved. Equally it would be dangerous for me to pretend a medical knowledge I do not possess and which might give false hope to others. I can only report my own case and the treatment I administered to myself and which has given me some 15 years' remission (if that is the correct term) for which I am profoundly grateful. I will resist describing a miracle panacea and merely record the facts as they were presented to me and which I acted upon. There are many cures being hawked around for every imaginable condition since alternative medicine captured the public's attention and we are entitled to a personal choice where our own health is concerned.

It happened like this: Nanette remembered what I had forgotten, namely that an old friend of ours, Roger MacDougall, a successful playwright (*To Dorothy, A Son*) and at one time a Professor of Logic at, I believe, UCLA, had also been struck down by MS. His

situation had been far worse than mine and eventually
he went blind and was confined to a wheelchair. His
friends used to go and read to him. Although blind and
immobilised, his brain was still as active as ever and he
applied logic to his plight, approaching it methodically
step by step.

First he took the mystery out of the name of the
disease. Multiple = many. Sclerosis = hardening. As he
understood it, the disease caused the sheath protecting
the nerves to be destroyed, leaving them bare like
electronic wires. Next he argued that if he cut his finger
the body's restorative powers grew new tissue over the
wound. Therefore, why wasn't the body able to repair
the damaged nerves? What attacked them in the first
place? He continued researching and discovered that
MS was virtually unknown in countries where the
staple diet was rice and maize. He then caused further
research to be undertaken and found that there was an
absence of gluten in rice and maize, whereas it was
present in wheat, barley, oats and rye. He put himself
on a gluten-free diet for a period of several years and
slowly his eyesight and general condition began to
improve, but the progress was too slow for his liking.
Although he had satisfied himself that the gluten
element in wheat, barley, oats and rye was a
contributory factor, by cutting them out entirely he had
also deprived himself of valuable trace minerals. So he
formed a company and began to produce a highly
potent vitamin supplement which he took with
concentrated B12. Again, this produced positive results
in his case. Anxious to share his good fortune, he wrote
several papers for scientific journals and immediately
ran into conflict with medical establishments on both
sides of the Atlantic. His findings were derided and
dismissed; he was threatened with prosecution if he
continued with his claims. Nevertheless, he persisted,
going underground as it were, and distributing a

pamphlet which described his own experience to anybody who asked for it. Staying within the law, he was careful never to solicit fellow sufferers, but equally never refused to share his experience with anybody who found their way to him for advice. What had started out as a personal mission became an obsession and he was determined not to be silenced. From that moment onwards, he devoted his entire life in an effort to convince the sceptical that what had happened to him through his own unaided efforts was at the very least worthy of a closer examination.

This, then, is the background to my own story.

Nanette tracked down Roger the day after the fateful pronouncement. At first she pretended she was ringing on behalf of a friend. Roger quickly saw through her subterfuge. 'Are you really talking about Bryan?' he asked. She broke down and confessed the truth. Roger immediately calmed her by saying, 'Well, dry your tears because your troubles are over. He's going to get better, no question about it. Throw all the medicines down the toilet and stop distressing yourself, otherwise we'll have you ill. Bryan's ill, but he's not going to die.'

The very next day he came to have lunch with us at Pinewood. I met a man nearing 70, bent but still sprightly, no longer blind and able to drive his car and, as he put it, 'run up the stairs'. He inspired immediate confidence and stated his case with measured emphasis, never exaggerating his claim, never promising an overnight miracle cure, but telling us how he had fought and overcome his own troubles and the troubles that came after. I am not somebody who scorns the enormous advances made in surgery and orthodox medicines, but even before meeting Roger I had always felt that there had to be other routes worth considering. If people want to go to faith healers, or take herbal cures, visit holy shrines, then good luck to them and they should not be mocked. I am not religious, nor did I turn to religion at this crossroads in my life. I listened to a man who spoke from bitter experience and decided that in the absence of any real aid from conventional sources, I could lose nothing by giving his regime a trial. He was not telling me to take any drugs, he was not selling me any magic potion and he wanted nothing in return. All that concerned and sustained him was a burning belief in his own life story. He was so quietly reassuring that I did not hesitate to test the diet he outlined. He provided Nanette with a book he had written and a diet sheet. I went back on the set after lunch with renewed hope.

For the next three years I stuck to his gluten-free diet supplemented by vitamins, together with daily doses of oil of evening primrose, which I continue to this day. I was also compelled to forego my favourite tipple, whisky, but was allowed a modest amount of wine, indeed any spirit that came from the grape. Nanette proved brilliant at finding palatable alternatives to my favourite foods and closely scrutinising every tin and packet for the forbidden ingredient before buying them. I can't say that my taste buds suffered one iota thanks to her dedication. It was as a result of her endless experiments that she came to write her first cookbook – *The Fun Food Factory* – designed primarily for children, which showed them there is life beyond junk food. It proved an enormous success and led to her having her own programme of the same name on London Weekend Television, and was followed up by a second book, *Fun Food Feasts*. So there was a pleasant aftermath to our initial troubles, and no more than she deserved. Throughout the first months of trial, I continued to direct *The Slipper and the Rose*, often working a 14-hour day and travelling long distances to the various locations. The film went on to be chosen as the Royal Command Film the following year. I found I had much more energy on the diet and can honestly report that I suffered no extra ill effect. Gradually my symptoms became less severe; I regained my balance and the aberration in my eyesight corrected itself.

I often think back to the traumatic period and shall never forget that first meeting with Roger MacDougall when he tore aside my layers of fear and ignorance and replaced them with hope. There was a stark contrast between the romance I was attempting to record on film and the backstage anguish that Nanette, much more than I, endured. Without her love and unwavering support, I doubt whether I would have lasted the course. I know that I could never have sustained my own resolve without her as we journeyed through unknown seas with only one map to guide us. I have met some remarkable women in my life as this account has noted, but nobody comes anywhere near my wife. She is not just a beautiful face: let anybody or anything threaten her family and she becomes a tiger not to be tangled with. Between us, we somehow managed to keep the secret from our two daughters and, with the exception of a handful of our closest friends, nobody suspected anything untoward.

Subsequently, I have undergone several insurance medical examinations when beginning other films, and naturally I have to disclose any past illnesses. When I reveal the MS diagnosis I am always told, 'Well, yes, there's no actual proof that a gluten-free regime helps. On the other hand, doesn't do any harm, I suppose. You have to realise the disease often goes into remission.' To which I say, I'll settle for remission that has lasted 15 years. I took no drugs, not even an aspirin, and have been able to keep up my usual punishing work schedule. I still get occasional pain when overtired and I have long since gone back to a careful, but normal, diet, semi but not rabidly vegetarian. Apart from the minor ills that all flesh is heir to, I seem to be holding together.

CHAPTER ONE

Vitamins, Minerals and Trace Elements

It is important to know that people following a diet and cutting out certain foods can deprive themselves of beneficial vitamins, minerals and trace elements, the shortage of which could be harmful. When gluten is being dropped from the diet, a definite substitute of certain vitamins is needed. Omitting milk could be harmful because of its animal fat content. In addition, it is a source of Vitamins B2, B12 and Calcium.

The best way of course is to eat other foods which contain these vital substances. However, one has to be very careful and as it is important for every Multiple Sclerosis patient to use certain vitamins, I would advise a supplement. In line with the Roger MacDougall programme, a very good formula was developed, which is as follows:

Choline Bitartrate 10.0 mg Vitamin B1 2.0 mg Vitamin B2 1.0 mg Vitamin B6 6.0 mg Vitamin C 25.0 mg Vitamin E 7.5 mg Folic Acid 0.015 mg Inositol 10.0 mg Nicotinamide 40.0 mg Calcium-D-Pantothenate 12.0 mg Calcium Glutonate 75.0 mg Magnesium Carbonate 75.0 mg Lecithin 25.0 mg

This formula is an important supplement in the treatment of Multiple Sclerosis, but these tablets and capsules should not, as is sometimes indicated, be seen as a cure for Multiple Sclerosis. They are a safeguard to supplement the altered diet, but many people feel that they give them a good source of energy.

The best way of course to supplement basic shortages of these vitamins is to take plenty of fresh fruit, fresh vegetables, natural foods and, to balance all this, a good intake of rice. Rice is an excellent remedy, called the yin and yang food in China. Here is a very good recipe.

Put whole brown rice in a casserole or a Pyrex dish. Pour boiling water over the rice and place the dish in a preheated oven. Cook it for 10 to 15 minutes and switch off the heat. Keep the rice in the oven for 5 to 6 hours. Cut up some vegetables such as parsley, chicory, celery and cress and mix this through the rice with a little garlic salt. Heat it up and the rice will be ready to use.

Do not underestimate the importance of a good balanced diet. Although these vitamins specified are made of 100 per cent biological natural ingredients and manufactured under strictly controlled conditions, it is nevertheless important that a healthy diet is taken care of.

As I have said before, one should see every Multiple Sclerosis patient as a completely individual case.

There is growing evidence in the United States that Multiple Sclerosis might be related to a virus, or to an allergy or even perhaps to an inherited problem. It is also known that if the cause were due to a virus, that virus remains in the wall of the small intestine. One of its products is super oxide radical. This radical is responsible for the destruction of the myelin sheath. The treatment plan based on this hypothesis is threefold.

Firstly, the virus must be removed from the body. This will be accomplished by using Interferon stimulance and immunoglobulins. Secondly, the super oxide radical must be removed, utilising the dismutation reaction. Thirdly, the physiological condition of the organ systems of the body must be restored to an optimum level.

Dr Harold Manner from the United States, with whom I work closely, has developed a schedule to be used in his clinics, which was printed for the practising physician. Added to this, however, was the warning that it should in no way be considered as a do-it-yourself manual. Professional diagnoses and regular checks are absolutely essential to the success of the treatment on this programme.

Vitamin and mineral levels of the Multiple Sclerosis patient are usually out of balance – it is therefore essential that the body be brought back to normal as rapidly as possible. Once vitamin and mineral deficiencies and surpluses are known, measures can be taken to correct the imbalance.

Although we know that Vitamin B complex is important to the Multiple Sclerosis patient, we should realise that Vitamin C is also of great importance. I have often come across improvement in the condition of Multiple Sclerosis patients after using Interferon. As this is sometimes difficult to obtain, we should remember that its production can be stimulated by Vitamin C. Hence the conclusion that a high dosage of Vitamin C for the Multiple Sclerosis patient can sometimes be beneficial.

By a dismutation reaction, the super oxide radical reacts with hydrogen under the influence of super oxide dismutase to produce hydrogen peroxide. This peroxide is then converted to water and pure oxygen under the influence of either peroxidase or catalase. This can be accomplished in the body by using dismutase tablets. However, I have found that using the mineral Germanium, which gives a boost release of oxygen, has been of great benefit to Multiple Sclerosis patients.

It is also important to stimulate the immune system. One can give Vitamin A in an emulsified form, which increases the number of circulating lymphocytes. Lymphocytes are additionally stimulated by the addition of thymosine, which will also help the immune system of a Multiple Sclerosis patient.

Vitamin E is essential to prevent oxidation of unsaturated fats and is also advised to be taken when on a gluten-free diet which excludes wheatgerms. Sometimes we advise patients to add a little extra Vitamin E to the amount which is recommended in the Roger MacDougall programme.

Vitamin F is also essential and is found in Oil of Evening Primrose, which is dealt with in a later chapter. When using Oil of Evening Primrose it is of great importance that Cod Liver Oil or a good fish oil is used to link up with this particular treatment.

One of the most important minerals for the Multiple

Sclerosis patient is Zinc. Some Multiple Sclerosis patients, who have a tendency to get depressed and downhearted, often benefit from additional Zinc. This mineral has the exceptional property of boosting the patient's morale when depression occurs.

Furthermore, we have Copper, Iron, Magnesium and Selenium – all of which minerals are found helpful in the total treatment of Multiple Sclerosis. Another much newer report is on Lecitone, which is a migration of lipid complexes in the body.

In order to better understand the efficacy of a dietary supplement based on dehydrated brain rich in brain lipid complexes, this migration in the body should be studied. This has been carried out more particularly with phospholipids which represent the essential of lipid complexes of the brain.

Mention must be made firstly of a publication of Gregoriadis who, in 1977, in *Life Sciences*, presented a remarkable summary of the biological role of lipid complexes. He noted that phospholipids are the essential constituents of intracellular biological membranes and that they are arranged in molecular layers characterised by a semi-liquid crystalline state. This physico-chemical characteristic being dependent upon the length and degree of unsaturation of the fatty acid chains, Gregoriadis emphasises the fragility of such membranes and the movements of phospholipid molecules. He explains phospholipid transfers occurring within a particular membrane, from one membrane to another and diffusions of exogenous phospholipids which are exchanged with damaged molecules. These findings led to the following conclusion: this dynamic state of phospholipids within or across cellular membranes as well as between cellular organelles is very relevant not only to the possibility of intercellular exchange of phospholipids but also to the mechanism of utilisation of exogenous phospholipids.

CHAPTER TWO

Oil of Evening Primrose

Evening Primrose is a small plant with bright yellow flowers which originated in North America. In the olden days Indians used it for medicinal purposes. It has been known for a long time that the extract of this little plant has great healing powers for skin conditions and is beneficial to the healing of infections.

Over 15 years ago this plant created a lot of interest. It was noticed that people who were using an extract from this plant healed more quickly after an operation than people who were not using it. Later, researchers looked into possible benefits for arthritis, skin and menopausal problems. Of course, in the present context, my main interest is in their findings relating to Multiple Sclerosis.

One might expect it to be a complex matter to find out exactly why the extract is beneficial but it contains one very important molecule, the gamma linoleic acid, or GLA as it is sometimes called, which is essential for health.

Many people have difficulty in converting linoleic acid into GLA. Oil of Evening Primrose has proven its value in providing people with health benefits which they otherwise would not possess. Most important is the conversion of linoleic acid into GLA. Until GLA is produced, it cannot be turned into the fatty acids which are vital to our health.

Linoleic acid is polyunsaturated and one of the most important substances in our food. This essential fatty acid, like vitamins, is necessary in the maintenance of a healthy body.

Most scientists have now come to the conclusion that linoleic acid plays a significant role in the prevention of all kinds of degenerative illnesses as well as heart diseases. Because of this, they realise the importance of Oil of Evening Primrose.

In this day and age there are many reasons why people get a deficiency of GLA. Convenience foods, hard margarine, certain biscuits, and products which are high in saturated fats such as butter, milk or red meat, can hinder the production of GLA in some individuals. It is also an accepted fact that serious illnesses, including cancer, can be caused by over-indulgence in alcohol. This creates deficiencies of several elements which cause the body to stop producing GLA.

In order to get the best benefit from Oil of Evening Primrose, researchers have found over the years that combining this oil with other vitamins and minerals enhances the health of the individual.

With a GLA content of 9 per cent, Oil of Evening Primrose is by far our richest source of this nutrient. Because this natural product can be used as a dietary supplement there is no problem using drugs. It does not force the body to do or produce anything but, as shown in recent research and tests by several scientists, it is almost unbelievable what this little yellow plant is capable of. Maybe not for every patient, but certainly for many, the improvements have been dramatic and it would be worth while to prescribe this extract, on trial for a lengthy period of time, to every Multiple Sclerosis patient.

In 1979, 480 Multiple Sclerosis sufferers took part in a particular survey while using Oil of Evening Primrose and it is heartening to learn that, of the participants, 65 per cent felt there was some improvement in their condition. Of these:

43 per cent thought there was a stabilisation in their condition;

22 per cent said they had suffered less severe attacks;

20 per cent felt an alleviation of particular problems;

13 per cent felt an improvement in their general health, and

2 per cent reported further beneficial side effects.

The full results were:

some improvement	65 per cent
no change	22 per cent
deteriorated	10 per cent
don't know	3 per cent

On a visit to South Africa in the mid-1980s, I interviewed quite a number of Multiple Sclerosis sufferers. Where Oil of Evening Primrose was used in combination with certain fish oils, a large majority reported surprising results.

During his research, my friend, Dr Hassam, found a shift in the proportion of saturated and unsaturated fatty acids recorded in the brains of Multiple Sclerosis patients. This was not totally unexpected, although results were inconsistent. This is often the result of a metabolic or nutritional disturbance during the period of brain growth, rather than during adulthood. Therefore, it is most important that nutrition, as discussed before, be taken into consideration while using remedies like Oil of Evening Primrose.

Luckily, taking these measures, a remission may be long standing or permanent. Of the various methods which are being used nowadays, this one seems to be most successful.

Unfortunately, the EFA – Essential Fatty Acids – are often ignored. One should never forget that fat is present in every cell of our body and that roughly 60 per cent of the structure of the brain is composed of fat. EFA is vital for the proper growth and development of the brain as well as the total nervous system.

In Multiple Sclerosis cases, the whole central nervous system is under attack. An unusual pattern of fatty acids has shown up in Multiple Sclerosis sufferers. By taking a diet rich in EFA, it was demonstrated that this pattern can be reversed within the period of one year. Even back in the 1970s, it was discovered that relapses were less frequent and that great successes were achieved in the rebuilding of the immune system when using sunflower oil.

Several laboratories have confirmed that Multiple Sclerosis

patients have a low concentration of Essential Fatty Acids, plasma, red blood cells and platelets in the nervous system.

To investigate this, a co-ordinated double trial, lasting two years, was set up in Belfast and in London. The diets of the Multiple Sclerosis patients were supplemented with either sunflower oil or olive oil and at the end of the trial it was found that relapses tended to be less frequent and that a better control was achieved by those on sunflower oil.

Professor Fields reached objective conclusions in his work and survey of Multiple Sclerosis. Further research is showing excellent results and will prove beneficial in the management of Multiple Sclerosis.

The dosage of Oil of Evening Primrose is variable. Personally, I prescribe four to six capsules per day. They are easily taken, and sometimes my advice is to gradually build up the dosage. Do not give up too quickly, but persevere, as it may take some time before effects are noticeable. People are often critical but, once they are interviewed, one discovers that they have only been using this extract for a short period of time.

A good capsule should contain not only Oil of Evening Primrose but also marine oil, so that with these two biologically active fatty acids, the right supplement is administered.

Occasionally, I have prescribed a higher dosage than normal, especially where I felt it desirable to speed up the process. Once I had a patient who told me why she really needed to see some improvement within the span of one year. I will end this chapter by telling you her story.

This patient was unable to walk and spent her life in a wheelchair. For some reason, she came to me convinced that I would be able to cure her overnight. I had to tell her that it is impossible to cure Multiple Sclerosis, but that it might be possible to control it.

I discovered that she had four sons, two of whom intended marrying the following year. I could not fail to notice the anxious look in her eyes when she told me that she wanted to walk out on that day, even if it was just in and out of the church. She assured me that she would do anything to achieve this.

I told her that I would treat her to the best of my ability and felt that a high dosage of Oil of Evening Primrose might show some results. She followed my instructions to the letter and, after some months, she was able to cross the streets in Glasgow where she lived, without any assistance. She did this much to the surprise of the policeman who was regularly on traffic duty there. He actually left his post for a moment to enquire what caused the improvement.

Mentally, this lady had been totally convinced that her condition could be improved, and she was committed to do anything within her power to help herself. She followed strictly and adhered to all the instructions given by me, but I still believe that the Oil of Evening Primrose was a great boost in this case.

I would recommend Multiple Sclerosis sufferers to try Oil of Evening Primrose as I have seen many cases in which it has been beneficial.

It has been of the greatest benefit for patients who use Oil of Evening Primrose to do this in combination with a capsule I use called PD Capsule. This is a protein deficiency formula which contains all the amino acids. The combination of PD Capsule and Evening Primrose works really very well and most patients report beneficial effects when using this combination.

CHAPTER THREE

Hyperbaric Oxygen

Sometime during the evening, after lecturing on Multiple Sclerosis in 1975 in Bienne, Switzerland, I was approached by Professor Dr Karl Asai from Japan, who has done a lot of research into the mineral Germanium. We had a very worthwhile conversation which continued well into the night.

Professor Asai has done much research on cancer patients, but he also noticed that Germanium had a good influence on those suffering from Multiple Sclerosis. One of the characteristics of the mineral Germanium is that it releases a lot of oxygen. Bearing this in mind, I have treated several patients with this mineral whenever I have been able to obtain it (as the process used to make it soluble is very intricate).

Almost miraculous results were obtained when I treated a Dutch patient of mine. I still doubt, however, that the diagnosis of Multiple Sclerosis in this patient was correct as she only displayed some symptoms peculiar to Multiple Sclerosis and no lumbar puncture was performed on her. Nevertheless, the fact remains that Multiple Sclerosis patients do react positively to Germanium. Consequently, when hyperbaric oxygen tests were established in Scotland, I followed their findings with added interest. I decided to try Germanium on some patients who came to me after having had several treatments in an oxygen chamber. Positive results showed in improvements of double vision, speech and bladder control.

During this test period, I was fortunate to meet Dr Ray Evers from the United States of America who has used a hyperbaric oxygen chamber in his clinic for many years. He told me that he once read an article entitled 'Is oxygen the missing piece in the ageing process and its related health problems?'. The article stated that even though water, juices, green juices and pure foods cleanse the body, unless there is an adequate supply of oxygen we have no solid foundation for life. A lack of oxygen in the system will prevent oxidation, which energises cells into a biological regeneration. The healing powers of oxygen have long been known. However, until the advent of hyperbaric oxygen – HBO – therapy, scientists were unable to uniformly introduce pure oxygen into the body's tissues.

Dr Evers began hyperbaric oxygen treatment in his health centre in Cottonwood, Alabama, in 1981. He found it an effective adjunctive therapy in the treatment of chronically degenerative diseased patients. He also told me that patients feel well after the treatment and that he did not discover any side effects. Treatment in a hyperbaric oxygen chamber is pleasant enough, but should always be administered by trained people.

Research has shown hyperbaric oxygen therapy to be an effective treatment, not only for Multiple Sclerosis, but also for people with other chronic degenerative diseases.

It depends totally on the patient how often treatments should take place. It is also very important that the atmospheric pressure to which the patient is subjected is carefully researched.

Under normal circumstances, oxygen is transported by haemoglobin, carried in the red blood cells. These cells are usually 98 per cent saturated with oxygen. However, the red cells constitute only about 45 per cent of the blood volume. Another carrier of O_2 is blood plasma. When the hyperbaric pressure is increased to two or more times the normal atmospheric pressure, the plasma becomes oxygen-rich to as much as 10 to 15 times its normal level. In fact, the plasma of patients receives enough oxygen to sustain life for a considerable period of time.

Dr Ray Evers also said that he did not claim hyperbaric oxygen treatment as a panacea for all chronic degenerative diseases. He has, however, seen dramatic results in many chronically degenerated patients who demonstrated oxygen deprivation. The guideline in the treatment of everything, from cancer to gangrene, is that the body is starved of oxygen, suffers poor circulation and is the unwilling victim of induced poisons and poor nutrition.

I am aware that Dr Evers has done a lot of valuable research over the years and for that reason I advised my patients to get in touch with the ARMS organisation for the treatment of hyperbaric oxygen now available in this country.

In an article written by Dr James from the Watson Institute, Dundee University, around 1985, I read that several ARMS centres had then been operative for over a year and many patients had been able to benefit from oxygen therapy. However, it also seems that patients and their families are confused about any relationship between the cause of Multiple Sclerosis and the use of hyperbaric oxygen.

Dr James states very clearly that Multiple Sclerosis is often described as a demyelinating disorder in which the myelin sheaths are separated from the nerve fibres. It is possible that some myelin sheaths may be reformed, although the evidence to date is that nerve fibres cannot be replaced. Often the myelin sheath acts as an insulator. In fact, the myelin sheath is present to increase the speed of conduction of the nerve impulse along the fibre.

Some of the facts show cause for optimism as it is proven that fat embolism can produce plaques in the human brain. These plaques are identical to those seen in established Multiple Sclerosis patients.

Patients known to have suffered from acute fat embolism can deteriorate in the same progressive way as Multiple Sclerosis patients. Fat embolism may therefore be one cause of Multiple Sclerosis, but it remains to be seen if it actually is the cause.

The clinical features of Multiple Sclerosis are entirely compatible with fat micro embolisms. Proof that the basic pathology in most Multiple Sclerosis patients is due to the fact embolism is difficult to provide, although there is massive circumstantial evidence.

It is therefore most important for everyone to realise that the use of hyperbaric oxygen in treatment does not require this proof, because the pathological features already established indicate that it is an agent of choice. Dr James came to these conclusions after excellent investigation on hyperbaric oxygen treatment. One of the most interesting things I read in this particular paper was that most drug treatments used for symptomatic therapy cause significant side effects. Oxygen is simply restoring the most favourable conditions for natural recovery.

In a worldwide test, about 3,000 Multiple Sclerosis patients were treated with hyperbaric oxygen, and the controlled studies proved its efficacy. Considerable improvement was obtained after exposure to HBO treatment – significant enough to carry on further testing.

A vital key for long life is that we carry an adequate supply of oxygen in our bloodstream. A continuous supply of oxygen is necessary to our survival and today, with constant atmospheric interference, it is important that we try to get out in the fresh air, sea air or mountain air, anywhere to get away from gases which are poisonous, and to fill our lungs with oxygen.

Our brains require oxygen to function properly, giving us more mental activity. We should never forget that the air consists of a mixture of 21 per cent oxygen, 78 per cent nitrogen and minor traces of other gases.

There are approximately 60 trillion cells in the human body and each cell is responsible for hundreds of chemical reactions to support life and requires the correct amount of nutrients and adequate oxygen. If the circulatory system is obstructed, many of these cells will starve from lack of oxygen, become diseased and will eventually die.

Breathing oxygen in cases of Multiple Sclerosis can sometimes affect improvement, but if the oxygen transport system is not functioning properly, hyperbaric oxygen treatment, in combination with Germanium, can improve the condition of a patient beyond belief.

The liver, which has to cope with influences from a variety of food and drink, suffers if its ally, oxygen, is not supplied in sufficient quantities to aid it with its intricate laboratory work. With many Multiple Sclerosis patients I have paid extra attention to the liver. This was mostly done with the help of some liver-cleansing products.

I constantly remind Multiple Sclerosis patients of the bad influence of alcohol and smoking, which really prevents them from improving their condition. Using Kirlian photography and comparing photographs which are taken before treatment with those taken after the diet is altered and smoking and drinking is cut down or out, significant differences are noticeable. One can see that the oxygen transport system is once more working normally.

It is important that Multiple Sclerosis patients take plenty of exercise and, in particular, do good breathing exercises to aid the transport of oxygen. Glycogen is a great source of energy, but it is limited by the amount of O_2 present. Oxygen therefore becomes a limiting factor, so it is important that enough is present for the effective use of glycogen.

Relaxation exercises in any form, especially when the Multiple Sclerosis patient is under stress, will always increase oxygen to the tissue cells. A decrease of oxygen will lead to the unavailability of oxygen to the lymphocytes which, in turn, will upset the hormonal balance supply of oxygen in the body.

Lymphocytes are normally contained in blood vessels. They leave the blood vessels to maintain the immunological balance of the body. Multiple Sclerosis patients lack oxygen and this decreases the ability in the brain and nervous system to patrol the tissue cells as they do in normal people. The nerve sheath will be gradually damaged in patients who suffer from lack of oxygen.

Eyesight often improves when a Multiple Sclerosis patient has hyperbaric oxygen treatment, because good eyesight depends on a good supply of oxygen in the blood.

All in all, we should realise that, whichever method is used, if one Multiple Sclerosis patient benefits, anything should be done to give other Multiple Sclerosis patients the chance to use this method. Any method should be available to every patient.

CHAPTER FOUR

Acupuncture

Frequently I am asked why I think that acupuncture works so well for Multiple Sclerosis patients. Harmony is one of the most important parts in the life of a Multiple Sclerosis patient. What impresses me always when I am in China is that the three important parts of the great temple in Peking are:

- the supreme temple
- the temple of perfection, and one would say that there is nothing better than perfection. For the Chinese, however, there is, because the third is
- the temple of harmony

This is acupuncture in a nutshell. Again, in this chapter, I will not go into great detail, but I just want to stress a few points, explaining why I am in favour of using acupuncture in the treatment of Multiple Sclerosis patients.

I often ask students to describe in their own words what illness is, and receive many different answers. Basically, illness is what the Chinese call 'disharmony'. We should aim at restoring harmony to that which has been out of harmony in the human body. In the case of Multiple Sclerosis patients, there can be quite a few disharmonies.

The Chinese made very sure of three things before I was ever allowed to touch a needle. I had to look, to listen and to feel. They are meticulous in their teaching of what to look for. Look how the hair grows, how the fingernails grow, how the ears stand, for instance. Then one learns to listen to the sounds the patient makes and, finally, one feels the patient.

What do we feel? Firstly, a good acupuncturist has to have a thorough knowledge of pulse diagnosis. It never ceases to surprise me that a very good Chinese acupuncturist will be able to tell how long a person has to live just by feeling their pulse.

Basically, what a good acupuncturist does is to ask himself, after having taken good note of the patient, where the energy in the patient is disturbed. Once we have made sure of our diagnosis, we look at the human body as a field of energy. Where disharmony is present, we are fortunate that, with the help of needles, we are often able to restore harmony. We have been taught which points to use, though sometimes a good acupuncturist follows his intuition. He will obtain good results by carefully choosing his points and using his capability as a therapist.

It has only happened once to me and might never happen again, but I will never forget a female Multiple Sclerosis patient, in her 30s, who was unable to walk and was bound to her wheelchair. After this patient was placed on the bench, I decided where the energy was disturbed and started with the treatment. Afterwards, she told me that she had some more feeling in her legs and when I asked her to try and stand, she managed to do so. During her next visit, I gave her more acupuncture treatment, this time choosing different points, and she managed to walk a little. She again told me afterwards that she felt a little better.

Over such a short period of time one cannot speak of a remission – but there definitely was a sudden change and restoration of energy. I was still sceptical about this sudden improvement, but had to believe it when, on her next visit, I did not see a wheelchair. When her name was called, she walked into my consulting room, happy and very much better. She remained very well until she was visited by a neurologist who told her that, although impressed with her improvement, he regarded it as only temporary. Of course, this depressed her totally and her husband, very upset, phoned to tell me that she had slipped back. I had a heart-to-heart talk with this lady and fortunately, after further treatment, she improved again.

This again proves that one should have a positive frame of mind no matter which treatment one receives or by whom the treatment is given. Especially when we talk in terms of energy, a positive mind is very important. This lady continued to feel well after her initial slip. I must add that an experience like this might happen only once in a lifetime, but nevertheless it is most encouraging. It also shows that we still know very little about energy.

During question time after lectures, I am often asked what the future of medicine is and generally my answer is that we are only scraping the surface as far as our knowledge of energy is concerned. In our present-day world, we need energy-giving foods and we need to learn to direct and transport energy. Anything which can aid a Multiple Sclerosis patient to do that is worth studying. This I often call the future of medicine.

Acupuncture, though often misunderstood, is an ideal method of restoring not only energy but also harmony to the human body. It is God's gift that these energy-restoring points have been discovered. Thousands of years ago, when the Chinese were fighting each other, they became aware of unexpected reactions when arrows hit certain points. This set their philosophers on the trail which resulted in the development of acupuncture. I am grateful that I have been able to benefit from such centuries-old knowledge and study.

In acupuncture, we use stomach points, spleen points, kidney points, bladder points and liver points, but it all depends on the symptoms of the Multiple Sclerosis patient concerned which points are relevant to his (or her) condition. With the present electro-acupuncture, very good results have been obtained by treating lung meridians, gallbladder, stomach and some of the governor points.

The auriculo-acupuncture therapy, which centres on the ear points, is useful in the treatment of muscles, joints, heel, toes, ankle, hip, shoulder and neck movements.

I have treated some Multiple Sclerosis patients suffering from leg spasms with electrical stimulation of several response points. This treatment, when followed up by auriculo-acupuncture, improved their voluntary motor control. This step-by-step programme has achieved some amazing results. It might be that these improvements are due to a change in the extra-cellular fluids, or it might be that the general condition of the patient greatly improved. Although there is still much research to be done, acupuncture used in cases of Multiple Sclerosis is invaluable.

Often I am told by Multiple Sclerosis patients who have been tense and stressed that after acupuncture treatment they feel much better. When the acupuncturist has assessed the imbalance, tensions can be released through use of needles in the chosen positions and gradual improvement for the patient should result.

Every human body has a built-in record of its own life history and all traumatic events leave a scar which can be systematically identified and sometimes interfered with surgically. Through restoration-acupuncture, some life forces can be released and a road to recovery may be found.

My friend and well-known doctor of acupuncture, Walter Thomson, once said in an important lecture that every action causes a reaction. He advised me at the time to use colour therapy in combination with acupuncture treatments. As colour affects us, like cosmic light affects the balance of life, I felt that he had given me good advice. For this reason, I occasionally use colour therapy in the treatment of Multiple Sclerosis. This can be carried out at home by the Multiple Sclerosis patient as it is possible to obtain a colour therapy apparatus. The programme to be followed is:

RED COLOUR

> The patient lies face down. Start at the base of the spine with magenta light (red and violet). Focus it on the Root Chakram for 15 minutes.
>
> Then slowly move it up the spine to the fifth dorsal

vertebrae – taking some five minutes to reach this part.

Focus on the soles of the feet for 15 minutes.

Each great sciatic nerve should be treated, allowing the light to play upon the back of the legs in an upward direction.

Change to red, treating the knees, shins and feet together for ten minutes.

Switch to indigo. Focus the light for five minutes upon the solar plexus.

Slowly move the indigo light up to the power centre in the throat. Focus it there for a further five minutes

Change to blue and green light for ten minutes.

If this programme for colour therapy is followed, the patient will feel better afterwards. We all know that light affects everything and it can be seen as the activator of life. Sensitivity to light for effectiveness by frequency of colour is an important factor.

As some Multiple Sclerosis patients have used methods such as shiatsu, acupressure or reflexology, I feel that perhaps this colour therapy should be fitted into that particular programme.

In acupuncture terms, it is most important to restore the yin and yang balance where it is disturbed, either anatomically or in other ways. It does not matter if the condition is chronic or acute, the uncomfortable problem is there and needs to be looked at. We are fortunate that this old and proven method is now getting more appreciation in our western world.

CHAPTER FIVE

Dental Care

The Toxicology Centre at the University of Tennessee is known as the best in the USA. In their evaluation of most toxic substances known to man, plutonium is listed as the most deadly, as it is lethal to humans in the least amount known. In an organic consumer report published by Eden Ranch I read that, on the rating scale used at the University of Tennessee, plutonium measures 1900+. Mercury, used in silver dental fillings, on the same scale measures 1600 and nickel measures 600.

Dr Willem Khoe has researched at length how much dental mercury or silver fillings are to blame for further damage to the health of Multiple Sclerosis patients. With the help of several case histories, he informed me that some of his Multiple Sclerosis patients have progressed well after these particular fillings were removed and replaced with composite fillings. This action was followed up with a homoeopathic antidote to mercury.

Since then, I have taken considerable effort to look into the effects of silver, mercury and nickel fillings. In my mind there is no doubt that, especially when the patients have an allergy, these fillings can influence their health detrimentally and might even be the cause of the ailment.

An explicit book, *How Safe are Silver (Mercury) Fillings?*, has been written by Betsy Russell Manning. The book is well researched and well referenced with numerous case histories. She has quoted some really astonishing cases and discussed the matter with dentists and psychiatric physicians.

One typical case concerns a 17-year-old girl who had changed from an outgoing, popular youngster with high school grades, to a recluse who refused to leave her mother's side. Asked to describe her daughter's behaviour, the mother explained that the girl suddenly reverted to speaking in a childlike manner and tone of voice and displayed an unnatural concern about death. Since the girl had already been seen by about 50 practitioners, including a cardiologist, internist, allergist, osteopath, gynaecologist, gyro-practitioner, psychiatrist and psychologist and had been hospitalised for tests, it cannot be argued that her treatment had not been submitted to the best and most expensive. Finally, a simple dental problem brought the girl into contact with a dentist who had researched symptoms of mercury toxicity. He thoroughly checked her past medical history and noticed that she had six small amalgam fillings.

Many symptoms have been dealt with in dental and medical papers and journals, singling out mercury, but none had mentioned silver-mercury fillings as a potential or suspected source. Once removal of the silver-mercury fillings was completed, a steady improvement was noticeable.

Until more dentists are aware of the problem, testing will still cause some difficulty as symptoms are not consistent in all patients. A general rule is to start with examination of the white blood count. Other monitored tests include blood chemistry profile, hair analysis for minerals, electro-cardiogram, body temperature, white cell morphological changes, urinary excretion of mercury, whole blood mercury levels, urinary Vit. C, specific gravity and Ph, electrical current (amperage) generated in the oral cavity and other noticeable changes. In some patients changes appear in all areas, but not always in consistent or predictable ways.

After removing dental amalgam fillings and washing mineral salts out of the system, some patients exhibit toxic reactions which have affected the peripheral nervous system, immune system and cardiovascular system. The mercury in the biological system appears to create or mimic many disorders in these three areas, which should be considered.

The report by Manning has given the medical profession something to think about and I am very pleased that in many parts of the world the problem is now receiving attention. Dentists are also taking action by researching into what extent these fillings can have a damaging effect on the general health.

Many years ago, when visiting Dr Issell's clinic in Germany, I wondered why he removed all teeth from serious cancer patients. He informed me that he wanted to eliminate in advance any effects of dental infection or of any fillings which might have a harmful effect.

In her book, Betsy Russell Manning talks about Dr Voll's system, which I have employed for a number of years, using acupuncture points in the toes and fingers to diagnose dental disease. As a result of this type of testing, it is possible to clear up dental problems which are related to the meridians or energetically to organs in the body.

One patient was also mentioned who was freed of his double vision after a wisdom tooth was extracted. Although this tooth was covered by a gold crown, the real problem was a silver filling underneath. After remedial action, this particular patient regained his normal vision.

One of my own patients improved greatly when I used a homoeopathic preparation which was made from a toxic substance and called a nosode for silver amalgam, which was diluted sixfold. After using this nosode, there was a reaction and I advised the patient to have her teeth checked thoroughly. One extraction was necessary, after which the expected improvement occurred.

Dr Voll has published a book in Germany in which he lists about 10 or 12 classic homoeopathic remedies to use alongside the nosode for amalgam. Using this method, some astonishing results were achieved.

Dr William Boericke, former Professor of Materia Medica of the University of California, San Francisco, has stated that every organ and tissue of the body is more or less affected by mercury. It transforms healthy cells into decrepit, inflamed and necrotic wrecks and decomposes the blood, producing a profound anaemia. The malignant force affects especially the lymphatic system with all its membranes and glands, as well as the internal organs and the bones. Even the mind may be affected with loss of memory and weakened willpower. The mouth's salivary secretions are increased, gums become spongy, recede and bleed easily, crowns of teeth decay, teeth loosen, feel tender and elongate.

Dr Willem Khoe, for whom I have great respect, once told me of a Multiple Sclerosis patient who came to see him. This patient had been advised that she had to learn to live with the problems of Multiple Sclerosis. When he examined her teeth, he came to the conclusion that he had to take her off all previous medication and had his dentist remove all old fillings. These were replaced by composite fillings. When the patient was asked for her comment on the treatment, she said that her energy level was up by at least 50 per cent since she began using the device to bring the upper and lower teeth into alignment. She felt that her energy drain had disappeared and that she was progressing all the time.

The fact that people suffer from Alzheimer's disease, which quite often is caused by aluminium poisoning, shows us that these tests cannot be ignored. I have learned that some universities in Great Britain are also seriously looking into this problem which, in cases of Multiple Sclerosis and other neurological problems, might be the cause or at least a contributory factor.

The Legislative Committee on Health Care in the United States is conducting a study on the Implants and Therapeutic Devices Disclosure Act. A proposal has been designed to establish the patient's right to know a doctor's responsibility to legislation.

At the 10th Yankee Dental Congress in January 1985, quite a few publications were presented dealing with a review of the present mercury diagnostic services. With some analyses and diagnostic tests, these proposals have been proven several times over.

I was asked to give a lecture in Toronto in March 1985, where

I was introduced by a pleasant gentleman, who said in his introduction that he felt that we had quite a few things in common. It was not until later that I learned that he was an American dentist who is greatly involved in this particular analysing work. He is part of the Amalgam Toxicity Diagnostic Services in Newton, USA, and has found several toxic effects in hydrargyrum mercury quicksilver, displaying itself in symptoms such as allergies, asthma, digestive disorders, skin eruptions, depression, tremors, paralysis, madness, cachexia, etc. Later, I listened to a very clear lecture he gave on this subject, from which I quote:

> The amalgam toxicity issue, which was dormant for a long time, has been revived again in the past few years. Most of us have been caught in the dilemma between the allegations of toxicity and the assurances of safety. It is a potentially explosive issue, which twice before deeply divided our profession. Mercury, the main ingredient of amalgam, is an element with many unique qualities; among others, it tends to polarise opinions.
>
> In conclusion, some of the obvious facts and verifiable facts:
>
> 1. Mercury is a metallic element with unique characteristics. One and a half times as heavy as lead, it is the only metal which is liquid at prevailing temperatures. Mercury evaporates readily, penetrates and dissolves all other metals. It is chemically active and combines eagerly with other elements, forming micro- and bivalent organic or inorganic compounds.
>
> 2. No living organism shows physiological need for mercury.
>
> 3. Mercury is inimical to life and for this reason it is used in antiseptics, disinfectants, pesticides, insecticides, preservatives, etc.
>
> 4. Mercury is toxic and should be handled with caution.
>
> 5. Dental amalgam is a mixture of metal alloy with mercury.

6. Amalgam fittings in the human mouth generate unphysiologic electrical currents.

7. Amalgam fillings in the human mouth release mercury vapour.

8. Elemental mercury can be converted to methyl-mercury by oral and intestinal micro-organisms.

9. Elemental mercury vapour and organic mercury compounds can penetrate tissue barriers.

10. Mercury accumulates in the body of mammals, including humans.

11. There is no linear correlation between the toxic effects of mercury and mercury concentration in blood, urine, or hair.

12. All the primary scientific research appears to indicate that amalgam fillings can be hazardous to health.

13. Diagnostic criteria used for the detection of macromercurialism are inappropriate for the diagnosis of micromercurialism.

14. Only valid scientific evidence of safety could possibly justify the continuation of amalgam use in dental practice.

I feel fortunate to have been able to meet Dr Victor Penzer, and a good relationship has developed between us. We are both trying to alleviate some of the suffering resulting from these unwanted problems.

CHAPTER SIX

Exercises, Drinking and Smoking

I was consulted by a Multiple Sclerosis patient who had attended our clinic regularly in the mid-1980s for about five or six years. With different methods she has been kept going, but she never shows any noticeable improvements. I know for a fact that it is her smoking which keeps her back from improving. She dislikes it intensely when, every time she consults me, I bring up the subject. It is a fact, however, that Multiple Sclerosis patients who smoke do themselves a lot of damage, not only by the nicotine poisoning, but also by endangering the supply of oxygen which is so vital, especially to those people.

With so many methods available today to assist smokers to kick the habit, there is no excuse. It is done so easily with the help of acupuncture treatment. The same day I saw that patient, I received a letter from another patient, which read: 'I want to thank you for the anti-smoking treatment. Instead of damaging my health, I have now saved enough money to go on a cruise and I am sure that I will not want to spoil the air of the Canary Islands with nicotine fumes which I now dislike intensely.' This particular patient had received acupuncture treatment and was happy, as most patients are, according to the many testimonials I receive. I would encourage anyone who smokes, to please seek help if you are not able to stop on your own. It is for the good of your health.

The same goes for the use of alcohol. Under the heading of Prologue – 'What You Can Eat', you have read that certain alcoholic drinks are allowed. Those are the ones which do not contain gluten. From what I have written in the chapter dealing with oxygen, we know that alcohol of any kind affects the liver, which is especially important in Multiple Sclerosis cases. I do know that when Multiple Sclerosis patients get depressed, it is so easy to be tempted, but please understand that with every alcoholic drink taken, you may delay any improvement which might be taking place. Surely it is not too great a sacrifice to give up. There are many other ways to combat depression.

One very much healthier way to achieve relief from depression is through exercise. This will keep you active and, at the same time, regulate the oxygen supply. Never underestimate the value of any exercises. In my book *By Appointment Only*, dealing with nervous disorders, I have described some very good breathing exercises which not only relax the patient, but stimulate the transportation of oxygen throughout the system.

In this chapter, I would like to mention some particularly good exercises for Multiple Sclerosis sufferers, developed by a Dutch colleague of mine who regularly contributes articles to a Dutch magazine specialising in Multiple Sclerosis. These exercises deal with the four main functions, i.e. sitting, standing, lying and moving.

Sitting – Let us first study the effects of the *wrong* posture when slumping in a chair:

> a. The head is hanging slightly forward, which decreases the flow of blood to the brain, thus reducing the oxygen supply. In this position, it is more difficult to think clearly or concentrate.
> b. Excessive tension is placed on the back of the neck and relaxes the throat area which is wrong.
> c. The thyroid gland is cramped.
> d. The chest is flattened, which complicates breathing.
> e. The back is rounded, which is unfavourable to the spine and causes extra tension on the back and lack of it on the front.
> f. Resting on the tail-end of the spine could eventually cause haemorrhoids.

g. Organs in the stomach are cramped and deep breathing becomes impossible.

h. When crossing the legs, the transport of blood is slowed down in the knee and only one foot is in touch with the ground.

i. Sitting with crossed arms also hinders breathing.

Now for the *proper* posture:

Sit in such a manner that the seat of the chair takes your total weight. Place both feet on the ground slightly apart. Pay attention to the position of the seatbones, which should be placed firmly on the seat of the chair.

Stretch the upper body and neck and reach with the crown of the head towards the ceiling, inclining the chin slightly towards the chestbone. Relax the arms and shoulders and rest arms on the thighs. Make sure the jaws are slack.

Feel the stomach to check if the breathing reaches down there.

Although it may sound complicated, in time this will become the natural posture. Of the four functions we are dealing with here, sitting should be considered the most important, as a large part of our lives is spent in this position.

To loosen the neck and shoulders, we gently and slowly do the following exercises:

1. Lean the head towards the right shoulder as if to touch the shoulder with the ear. Do not raise the shoulder, but keep it relaxed. Repeat twice.

2. Make as if to wipe the ear over the shoulder. Repeat twice.

3. Again incline the head towards the right shoulder. Drop gently forwards, move towards the left shoulder and drop the head back, thus making a circular movement with the head. Repeat twice.

4. Repeat these three exercises to the left.

5. Breathing in, drop the head back; breathing out, drop it forwards.

6. Stretch the vertebrae of the neck while shoulders are still relaxed. Look over right shoulder and turn to face forwards. Repeat twice and do same exercise on the left three times.

After these neck exercises, we now concentrate on the shoulders:

1. Pull up the right shoulder as high as possible and then lower. Repeat twice.

2. Bring right shoulder horizontally forwards and then backwards without pulling the shoulder up. Repeat twice.

3. Repeat these exercises towards the left.

Standing – Stand up with the feet slightly apart. Position the feet in direct line with the hips. Relax the knees and place feet firmly on the ground. Achieve the correct position for the pelvis by straightening the spine and stretching the neck.

Make your arms hang down heavily so that the shoulders are relaxed. Jaws also should be relaxed. Oddly, tight jaws may produce tension in the stomach area. Keep the stomach relaxed to facilitate free and easy breathing.

Now we do the 'elephant wobble'. Shift the weight from the left to the right leg. In this way both legs relax in turn.

Rhythmic movements always have a relaxing effect. With the hips, gently make the figure-eight movement sideways.

To strengthen the hips, place the feet firmly on the ground and reach upwards with either arm in turn as if picking fruit which is just within reach. Follow this movement through with the hips.

The following little exercise goes to improve our instinctive breathing pattern. Stretch one arm forward and return the arm to the side of the body. Repeat this movement changing arms every now and then. Note that we breathe in when stretching and breathe out when retracting the hand.

Lying – Make sure there is plenty of room in order to be comfortable. When lying in a cramped position, the transportation of oxygen is hindered. Take up a position on your back with the arms slightly removed from the body, hands and fingers relaxed, feet again slightly apart and in line with the hips. Some prefer to have a small cushion under their knees, the waist or the head. Make yourself comfortable and be aware of all the areas of your body which touch the floor: the heels, calves, thighs, bottom, back, shoulders and finally the head.

Take deep breaths. Move fingers, toes and stretch hands and feet. Make a fist.

Stretch various parts of the body and yawn.

Slowly pull up the right knee so that the sole of the foot is flat on the ground. Feel the change in the back. Then pull up the left knee. Place right hand under the left knee and left hand under the right knee at the back of the thighs (thumbs on the inside and fingers on the outside). Pull your knees up towards the body and gently rock with small movements from left to right. Repeat these movements many times while gradually extending the movement.

At the end of these lying exercises, slowly pull up into a sitting position. Take your time to come out of this relaxed state.

Moving – The same rules apply here as for standing. Models learn to walk properly by balancing a book on their heads. After practice, they don't need the book any more: thinking of the book will be enough. Again breathe with awareness.

Another wonderful way to help the condition of Multiple Sclerosis sufferers is with the old method of cold washing. It is recommended to develop the habit of cold-water washing immediately on rising in the morning. Cold water stimulates the blood circulation and the body's activities. Never use warm water when bathing. However, the body and surroundings should be warm when taking a cold bath or shower, thus the body will react to the warmth.

One should acclimatise gradually to this treatment and begin with rubbing the body down with cold, wet towels first, starting from the top rubbing downwards. A cold bath or shower should never last longer than one minute. Warm water slackens the skin, while cold water spurs it on to activity.

Hydrotherapy is also advantageous in helping defective circulation. A long time back Father Kneipp gave us many good methods of hydrotherapy. I found that a simple way of improving the circulation was a method I learned from an old Indian doctor. This is part of my recommended treatment for Multiple Sclerosis and I refer to it as the 'Cold Dip'.

This exercise should be done each morning on rising and each night on retiring. Place a basin of cold water with a towel at the side of the bed. On rising in the morning, place both feet into the water and count to ten. Then place the feet on to the towel and exercise the toes as if trying to pick up a marble. Do this 10 to 30 times. On retiring, carry out the same exercise and you will find that your feet are as warm as toast when you get into bed. It is important that this exercise should be kept up for a minimum of 60 days if you want to feel the benefit. It may look simple but, if carried out properly, will have a remedial effect.

One patient came to me after doing this therapy for a little while and was so enthusiastic that he had almost made up his mind that this would help him to solve his problems. Sometimes we see this euphoria with Multiple Sclerosis patients and it could be looked on as a blessing in disguise. Somehow this euphoria helps to carry the patients through the problems of their disease. It also must be a help to their relatives. Patients with euphoria are usually cheerful, bright and appear happy with their lot in life. They talk a lot, laugh and generally seem happy, despite their physical incapacities and, to look at them, you wonder what they have to be cheerful about. Perhaps this is God's way of helping to cope.

Despite this exaggerated feeling of well-being in his patients, the practitioner should not underestimate the fact that all treatments should be directed carefully and a proper control of the patient has to be exercised.

Multiple Sclerosis patients could be divided into two groups. One group has this positive and sometimes euphoric feeling, while the other often feels depressed and miserable, making it difficult for the family to cope. Fortunately, the euphoric patients tend to approach things in a positive manner and, because of this, will benefit from the exercises.

In my opinion, one of the finest exercises has been designed by Dr H. Moolenburgh from the Netherlands on the basis of the Simonton approach.

First Part – Sit down in an easy chair, with your head resting, your feet flat on the floor. Breathe calmly and hear your breath going in and out. Now take a very deep breath and, when exhaling, say to yourself – Relax! Do this three times.

Now you are going to relax all the muscles of your body. Begin with your eyes and mouth. Squeeze your face tightly together and then suddenly let go. Feel a wave of relaxation travel down your body. Relax consciously your neck, shoulders, arms, hands, stomach, back, upper legs, calves and feet. When you have done this, try to remember a pleasant spot where you would like to be – a lake, a mountainous area, just some holiday spot of which you have fond memories. Imagine you are there and stay with the memory for a couple of minutes. This is the preparation for the main part of the exercise.

Second Part – Now you are going to *see* your illness. You are going to *see* with your mind's eye your spinal cord and in this white glistening cord you *see* some inflamed patches. Sort of gloomy, grey patches that do not look bright, and you are going to *see* with your mind's eye how the bodily defences deal with them. You *see* blood vessels opening, bringing a flood of healthy blood loaded with vitamins. You *see* building cells, restoring your fatty layer around the nerve track. If you want to imagine the thing as electric wires being restored, with new insulation being put around them, it is all right. As long as you *see* with your mind's eye how, with the help of vitamins, minerals and the body's own defence system, the spinal cord is restored to its old function.

Now, when you have finished this mental picture (and you

may use your own imagination, as long as you see your illness as *weak* and your bodily defence as *strong*), you are going to *see* yourself quite strong again. You *see* yourself walking normally, full of vitality. Pat yourself on the back for having done so well. Breathe deeply three times. Open your eyes.

Do this exercise three times a day: when you wake up, at lunchtime and before you go to sleep. Be in a quiet room. Never skip an exercise. Do not force yourself, just *see* it with your mind's eye. That is enough. What you are really doing is putting a new (and healthy) programme into the computer. It may take up to 6 to 12 months before the new programme starts to work out in your body.

Another good way to help the Multiple Sclerosis patient is the Alexander technique, which is a fresh approach to treatment. It cares for the maintenance of health in many conditions classed as neurological disorders, which are given a hopeless prognosis. Even problems like muscular dystrophies and those associated with a repeated trauma, where patients become accident-prone and more off-balance, benefit from the Alexander technique.

It is aimed at the realignment of the body framework to the adverse conditions. It is reported that wheelchair cases, who have to exert so much effort to do the simplest of things, have shown great improvement after having practised the Alexander technique. I do feel that if there is an interest in the Alexander technique, the Multiple Sclerosis patient, who usually has the time to do all these exercises, would benefit.

I totally disagree with the often repeated statement that exercises and physiotherapy will do no good for Multiple Sclerosis sufferers. Many benefit, for example, from yoga exercises. I have had a running battle with the UK National Health Service about physiotherapy treatment being made available to Multiple Sclerosis sufferers. It is said too often that it is a lost cause and that nothing can be done any more. The Health Service should provide these methods to Multiple Sclerosis sufferers.

Please take every opportunity to exercise and if your doctor is kind enough, I am sure he will do his best to produce physiotherapy treatment. Plenty of good books are written on the subject of yoga and these exercises should also be given consideration.

Finally, I would like to mention osteopathy. Although I have practised osteopathy for more than 25 years, I do not want to go too deeply into this subject, but one thing always comes to the fore. With every Multiple Sclerosis patient, I find that the third and fourth cervical vertebrae need adjusting. A good osteopath should be consulted and from time to time the spine should be manipulated.

Generally, I find that a spinal dorsal five adjustment will give relief and also that the dorsal 12 should be seen to for correct adrenaline supply. From time to time, a good massage is beneficial for the circulation. One should, however, be careful with reflexology, that not too much excitement is aroused, especially when the Multiple Sclerosis patient has muscular spasms.

With all the alternative techniques which are available, there is hope for Multiple Sclerosis sufferers that, by practising some of these methods, their condition will improve.

CHAPTER SEVEN

Eating your Way to Better Health

It is of constant annoyance for the MS patient to see how difficult the gluten-free diet can be, because of taste and even smell. Over the years that I have treated MS patients, they all keep moaning how tasteless their food can be. This is not always true because a lot can be done to improve the taste.

Jayne Martin, who was very obedient when it came to dietary restrictions, started on a discovery path on what could be done and, therefore, the recipes and common sense that Jayne has put into this book will be of the greatest help to MS patients.

It has also become more and more recognised how important diet is. I remember that Roger MacDougall and I went to a university here in Britain to plead for the understanding of his dietary management. During that conversation, schizophrenia and autism came up. Roger said then at that meeting – and that was well over 18 years ago – how he saw that, with some schizophrenics, the diet was helpful, but this was especially so with autism. After that statement when we pleaded with this professor of nutrition, he very kindly led us to the door, and I am quite sure that he thought we were a couple of nutcases. We then went to another university, this time pleading for the removal of dental amalgam. I am very sorry that Roger MacDougall never read the tremendous statements made by some universities, especially from the United States, on how the removal of gluten from the diet of autistic children has given such great results, and the scientific back-up of what we then said more than 18 years ago is approved of by many today.

The world has changed and diet is very, very important. It is therefore of great importance that the MS patient is prepared to follow this system which has been proven to be of great help to so many and, by adhering to the rules of the dietary management fully, should have success. I personally see that patients do get results when they follow the advice conscientiously, and therefore I am happy with the tremendous dietary advice that Jayne has given for this book. With her help, a lot more variation can be made to the diet and hopefully make the life of MS patients a little better. Certainly her recipes will add a lot of taste to the daily dietary management of the MS patients. This is Jayne's story.

'Since November 1991, I have experienced from time to time a variety of symptoms which I have been advised have been caused by an attack upon the nervous system. Whatever I may suffer from, I was determined not to accept my condition "lying down".

'Because Multiple Sclerosis appeared to be a possibility, I took great interest in discovering how others had fought the symptoms. My enquiries led to a friend who provided me with the address of the office of Mr Bryan Forbes. I have read his book, *A Divided Life*, and I was interested to discover that Mr. Forbes followed a particular diet. His secretary forwarded to me a booklet written by Professor Roger MacDougall and its contents have had a profound effect upon me. I was deeply impressed by his remarkable and successful fight to control his Multiple Sclerosis symptoms by following a strict dietary regime. I had received no advice in that connection but was determined to follow this regime.

'The vitamin/food supplement as formulated by Roger MacDougall I discovered could be obtained, by great coincidence, from Regenics, Wheelton, Chorley, Lancashire, which is virtually round the corner from my home. A further stroke of good fortune for me was to discover that Jan de Vries held a monthly clinic at the premises of Regenics. From his advice in consultation, I was more than ever determined to follow a particular diet. Problems then presented themselves. I had to set about the task of where best to obtain the necessary ingredients and recipes for my purpose. For instance, I did not know that soy sauce contained gluten. However, I now know that Meridian Foods Ltd. make gluten-free soy sauce (obtainable from most health food stores).

'It has taken some time and effort to gather the information now contained in this part of the book. I found that the search added to the general stress I was then undergoing and, therefore, considered that the information collated might be of some use to others who would wish to follow a similar diet. The contents of the book will also assist others who cannot eat products which contain gluten or have an illness which will not tolerate it. I now feel completely well again and I dedicate this part of the book to Jan de Vries.

Jayne Martin

Contents

Conversion Tables
Soups and Starters
Miscellaneous
Chicken Dishes
Meat Dishes
Oriental Section
Fish Dishes
Cakes and Bread
My Useful List
Things You Can Eat

Conversion Tables

Weights		Volume	
½ oz.	10 g	2 fl. oz.	55 ml
¾ oz.	20 g	3 fl. oz.	75 ml
1 oz.	25 g	5 fl. oz. (¼ pint)	150 ml
1 ½ oz.	40 g	10 fl. oz. (½ pint)	275 ml
2 oz.	50 g	1 pint	570 ml
2 ½ oz.	60 g	1 ¼ pints	725 ml
3 oz.	75 g	1 ¾ pints	1 litre
4 oz.	110 g	2 pints	1.2 litres
4 ½ oz.	125 g	2 ½ pints	1.5 litres
5 oz.	150 g	4 pints	2.25 litres
6 oz.	175 g		
7 oz.	200 g	Dimensions	
8 oz.	225 g	¼ inch	5 mm
9 oz.	250 g	½ inch	1 cm
10 oz.	275 g	¾ inch	2 cm
12 oz.	350 g	1 inch	2.5 cm
1 lb.	450 g	2 inches	5 cm
1 lb. 8 oz.	700 g	4 inches	10 cm
2 lb.	900 g	6 inches	15 cm
3 lb.	1.35 kg	7 inches	18 cm
4 lb.	1.8 kg	8 inches	20 cm

OVEN TEMPERATURES

Gas Mark	Fahrenheit	Centigrade
1	275	140
2	300	150
3	325	170
4	350	180
5	375	190
6	400	200
7	425	220
8	450	230
9	475	240

Soups and Starters

MELON AND GRAPEFRUIT COCKTAIL
1 melon
3 grapefruits
raw cane sugar

Peel grapefruits and remove pith. Cut melon into bite-sized pieces. Mix well and sprinkle with raw cane sugar. Leave until sugar has dissolved.

This can be frozen.

WATERCRESS AND POTATO SOUP
2 bunches of watercress
¾ pint goats' milk or other milk
¾ pint chicken or vegetable stock
¾ lb potatoes
1 onion

Sauté the watercress, potatoes and onion for 2 minutes. Add stock and milk and simmer for 25 minutes. Add salt and freshly ground pepper. Purée using blender or food processor.

This can be frozen.

LENTIL SOUP
1 tbsp sunflower oil
2 carrots, peeled and diced
1 medium onion, peeled and chopped
1 medium stick celery, trimmed and thinly sliced
2 cloves garlic, peeled and crushed
8 oz red lentils, rinsed
14 oz tin chopped tomatoes
1 bay leaf
2 pints vegetable stock
½ level tsp salt and freshly ground black pepper

Heat the oil in a large saucepan. Stir in carrots, onion, celery and garlic and fry for 5 minutes over a moderate heat.

Add the lentils, tomatoes, bay leaf and stock. Bring to the boil, then reduce the heat, cover and cook gently for about 40 minutes or until the lentils are tender. Discard the bay leaf. Season with salt and pepper.

MINESTRONE SOUP
1 onion
2 carrots
2 courgettes
1 leek
6 oz cabbage
small tin sweetcorn (without sugar)
14 oz tin chopped tomatoes
2½ pints vegetable stock
1 tube tomato purée
2 bouquets garnis
4 cloves garlic
4 oz gluten-free pasta spirals or other pasta
little sunflower oil

Fry the onion and garlic for 2 minutes.

Add finely diced carrots, courgettes and leek and cook for

about 10 minutes until soft. Add the stock, purée and tomatoes, shredded cabbage, sweetcorn and bouquets garnis. Bring to the boil. Add the pasta spirals and simmer for 20 minutes.

TOMATO SOUP
2 lb ripe tomatoes
1 large onion, chopped
1 large potato, chopped
1 clove garlic (optional)
¾ pint stock
drop sunflower oil

Gently heat the oil in a pan. Add onion and potato and fry for a couple of minutes, but do not brown.

Pour boiling water over tomatoes and leave for a couple of minutes. The skins will then come off quite easily. Chop the tomatoes and add to the pan containing the onion and potato. Add stock and simmer for about 25 minutes. Blend or put in a food processor.

Miscellaneous

OVEN-ROASTED RATATOUILLE
2 medium courgettes
1 small aubergine
1 lb ripe Italian plum tomatoes or any other red tomatoes
1 small red pepper, deseeded and cut into 1 inch squares
1 small yellow pepper, deseeded and cut into 1 inch squares
1 medium onion, peeled and chopped into 1 inch squares
2 large cloves garlic, finely chopped
1 packet fresh basil leaves or dried equivalent
1 heaped tsp crushed coriander seeds
3 tbsp olive oil
salt and freshly ground black pepper

Dice courgettes and aubergine into 1 inch squares. Place them in a colander and mix them with one rounded dessertspoon of salt. Then place a plate on top of them and weigh it down with a heavy weight making sure you have plate underneath the colander to catch the drips. Leave for about 45 minutes. Pour boiling water over the tomatoes and leave them for 1 minute. Drain, slip the skins off and quarter. When the aubergines and courgettes have drained, squeeze out any excess juice, then dry them thoroughly in a clean cloth. Preheat oven to highest setting. Now arrange tomatoes, aubergines, courgettes, peppers and onion on a roasting tray. Sprinkle with the garlic, chopped basil leaves, crushed coriander seeds and pepper. Drizzle the oil over, then mix thoroughly to give a good coating of oil. Roast on the highest shelf for 30–40 minutes or until the vegetables are tender and tinged brown at the edges.

FETA AND MUSHROOM RISOTTO
2 tbsp oil
1 onion, peeled and finely chopped
2 cloves garlic, peeled and crushed
2 large flat mushrooms, wiped and sliced
8 oz risotto rice
3 oz sun-dried tomatoes in oil, drained and chopped
1½ pints vegetable stock
2 oz feta cheese, cut into small cubes
salt and freshly ground black pepper
squeeze lemon juice
fresh chives, snipped, to garnish

Heat the oil in a pan and fry onion and garlic until softened. Add mushrooms and stir around for a minute. Add rice and sun-dried tomatoes and stir to mix. Pour over a little stock and bring to the boil. Simmer until stock is absorbed, then add a little more. Continue like this until all the stock is used up and the rice is tender. Add cubed feta at the end of cooking. Season with freshly ground black pepper and a little salt if necessary. Add a squeeze of lemon juice. Sprinkle with snipped chives to serve.

RICE WITH SUMMER VEGETABLES
8 fl. oz long-grain rice
3 small courgettes
2 red or yellow peppers
2 sticks celery
4 oz mangetout
1 large clove garlic
2 spring onions
2 tbsp extra virgin olive oil
¼ tsp powdered cinnamon

2 fl. oz dry white wine
1 tbsp lemon or lime juice

Cook rice until just cooked, not overcooked. Pour into a sieve and rinse under the cold tap until fully cooled, then leave to drain. Meanwhile, wash and trim the courgettes, peppers, celery and mangetout and cut into bite-sized pieces. Finely chop the garlic. Trim the onions and cut into fine shreds. Heat the oil gently in a large frying pan or wok. Add the cinnamon and garlic, stir to mix well, then add the chopped vegetables with some salt and freshly ground black pepper. Stir-fry over a medium heat for 2–3 minutes. Pour in the wine and continue frying until most of the liquid has evaporated. Add the rice and spring onions, then turn down the heat and stir-fry for 3 minutes. Stir in the lemon or lime juice.

YOGHURT SALSA
3 tbsp minced red onion or spring onion
1 tsp minced ginger
1 tsp minced green chilli with the seeds removed
2 tbsp minced fresh coriander
1½ tbsp lemon juice
4 fl oz bio or Greek yoghurt

Mix all the minced ingredients with lemon juice and season with salt and freshly ground black pepper. Leave this for at least 15 minutes. Immediately before serving, add the yoghurt and mix well.

EGG AND VEGETABLE BAKE
2 oz leek or celery, sliced
2 oz carrot, thinly sliced
2 oz onion, thinly sliced
½ small clove garlic, finely chopped
7½ oz tin chopped tomatoes

¼ tsp chopped fresh rosemary or pinch of dried rosemary
3 oz cooked kidney beans
1 medium-sized egg
½ oz half fat Cheddar cheese, grated
salt and pepper

Put the leek or celery, carrot and onion in a small saucepan. Stir in the garlic, tomatoes, herbs and seasoning. Cover and simmer gently for about 25 minutes until the vegetables are tender, stirring occasionally. Add the beans and cook for a further 2 minutes. Turn mixture into a small ovenproof dish, make a hollow in the centre and break in the egg. Season and sprinkle over the cheese. Cook under a moderately hot grill for about 5–10 minutes or until egg is cooked. Serve at once.

Chicken Dishes

CANNELLINI CHICKEN
4 pieces chicken
2 medium onions
1 green pepper
1 tbsp paprika
½ pint chicken stock
2 tbsp tomato purée
7½ oz tin tomatoes
marjoram or oregano
oil for cooking
salt and pepper
15 oz tin cannellini beans
Preheat oven to 180°C/350°F/Gas mark 4.

Brown the chicken in oil gently, then transfer to casserole. Using the pan in which the chicken was browned, fry the onions and pepper until shiny. Add the paprika and stir, then add tomatoes, tomato purée and stock. Finally add the marjoram or oregano, salt and pepper.

Place in the casserole and cook for 1 hour. Add beans 15 minutes before end of cooking time.

CHICKEN MARENGO
4 chicken breasts
14 oz tin tomatoes
1 or 2 medium onions
tin tomato purée
½ lb mushrooms
oregano or mixed herbs
cornflour to thicken if necessary
salt and pepper
glass white wine (optional)

Cook chicken and onion in small amount of oil for a couple of minutes. Add tin tomatoes, salt and pepper and simmer gently for 30 minutes, then add tomato purée, mushrooms, herbs, wine and drop of water. Simmer for further 5 minutes, ensuring chicken is thoroughly cooked. Thicken with cornflour, if necessary.

CHICKEN CASSEROLE
(suitable for quick, easy cooking in the microwave)
4 chicken quarters
1 onion, diced
2 carrots, sliced
1 pepper (or ½ green and ½ red), sliced
6 oz mushrooms, sliced
2 tbsp tomato purée
¾ pint chicken stock
seasoning
fresh herbs
cornflour for thickening, if necessary
oil for cooking

Remove skin from chicken quarters and toss in seasoned flour. Heat the oil for 40–60 seconds in a large casserole dish. Add chicken pieces and cook for 5–6 minutes, turning once during the cooking cycle.

Remove chicken from dish. Add the vegetables to the casserole and cook for 5 minutes. Add tomato purée and any remaining flour. Stir well and cook for 1 minute. Remove the casserole from the oven and gradually stir in the chicken stock to avoid lumps occurring. Return to the oven and cook for 2–3 minutes, stirring twice.

Add chicken to casserole and continue cooking for 10–15 minutes until chicken is tender and cooked. Check seasoning.

Serve with minted new potatoes or rice.

CHICKEN IN BARBECUE SAUCE
8 small chicken joints
Sauce
1 medium onion, finely chopped
1 large or 2 small cloves garlic, crushed
1 tbsp natural cane sugar
5 tbsp dry cider (or wine)
5 tbsp gluten-free soy sauce
1 heaped tbsp tomato purée
1 heaped tbsp mustard powder
olive oil
freshly ground black pepper
Preheat oven to 200ºC/400ºF/Gas mark 6.

Pat chicken with kitchen paper, ensuring it is absolutely dry, then rub each joint with olive oil and season with freshly ground black pepper. Pop them in a shallow roasting tin, tucking the chopped onion amongst them, and sprinkling them with a few drops of oil. Place on highest shelf and cook for 30 minutes.

To prepare the sauce, crush the garlic clove and add the rest of the ingredients to it. Whisk with a fork until blended thoroughly. When the chicken has been cooking for 30 minutes, pour off any excess oil from the tin and pour the sauce over it. Cook for a further 25 minutes, basting frequently.

Serve with brown rice and salad.

CHICKEN RISOTTO
4 chicken breasts, skinned and cubed
2 tbsp sunflower oil
1 red pepper, deseeded and diced
1 medium onion, sliced
1 garlic clove, crushed (optional)
3 medium carrots, peeled and sliced
4 oz mushrooms, sliced
8 oz brown rice
1 pint chicken stock
4 oz frozen peas
2 tbsp mixed herbs

Fry chicken in the oil for 4–5 minutes. Add onion, garlic, carrots, mushrooms and pepper and fry for a further 2–3 minutes until softened. Add rice, stock, peas and herbs. Bring to the boil, cover and simmer for 30–35 minutes, stirring occasionally. The rice should absorb all the liquid. However, if after the cooking time there is a little liquid left, remove lid and boil excess away. If risotto becomes too dry, add a little water to prevent sticking.

CHICKEN AND MUSHROOM FRICASSEE
4 oz skinned and boned chicken breast
1 oz sliced onion
1 oz sliced carrot
thin slice lemon
pinch dried mixed herbs
salt and pepper
2 oz sliced mushrooms
1½ tsp cornflour
4 tbsp skimmed milk
1 tsp chopped fresh parsley

Place chicken in a small pan. Add onion, carrot, slice of lemon, mixed herbs and seasoning. Add ½ pint cold water. Bring slowly to the boil, cover and simmer for 30 minutes. Add mushrooms and continue to cook for a further 5 minutes or until chicken is tender. Drain, reserve stock and discard lemon slice. Cut chicken portion into cubes or slices.

Blend cornflour with milk and make up to ¼ pint with reserved chicken stock. Pour into pan and bring to the boil, stirring, then add parsley. Return chicken and vegetables to sauce and heat through for about 2 minutes. Adjust seasoning.

SPANISH-STYLE RICE WITH CHICKEN
1 tbsp sunflower oil
1 onion, sliced
2 cloves garlic, crushed
½ tsp turmeric
4 skinless and boneless chicken thighs, cut into chunks
4 oz frozen peas
12 oz packet cooked, mixed seafood
10 oz long-grain white rice
1½ pints chicken stock
1 red pepper, deseeded and diced
4 oz mushrooms, sliced

Heat the oil in a large pan and fry the onion and garlic until soft. Add the turmeric and fry for 1 minute. Add the chicken and fry for a further 2–3 minutes to brown on all sides.

Add the rice and cook for 2 minutes. Pour the stock over and cook, stirring occasionally, for about 15 minutes. Stir in the red pepper, mushrooms and peas and cook for a further 10 minutes or until the liquid is absorbed and the rice is tender.

Add the packet of cooked seafood and heat through thoroughly for 5 minutes.

Serve hot.

INDIAN-STYLE CHICKEN
4 chicken breasts, skinned
5 oz natural yoghurt
1 onion, chopped
3 cloves garlic
2 bay leaves
2 tbsp lemon juice
2 tsp ground turmeric
2 tsp ground cumin
2 tsp ground ginger
2 tsp ground coriander
1 tsp mild chilli powder
salt and pepper
Preheat oven to 230°C/450°F/Gas mark 8.

Blend all the ingredients (except the chicken) in a large bowl.

Place the chicken breasts in the marinade for 24 hours. Place chicken into an ovenproof dish and cover with yoghurt mixture. Season with salt and pepper. Bake in a preheated oven for 30 –40 minutes.

HARLEQUIN CHICKEN
6 chicken portions, cut into bite-sized cubes
1 small red pepper, halved and deseeded
1 green pepper, halved and deseeded
1 small yellow pepper, halved and deseeded
1 small onion, thinly sliced
14 oz tin chopped tomatoes
2 tbsp fresh parsley, chopped
freshly ground black pepper to taste
1 tbsp sunflower oil

Cut the peppers into small diamond shapes.

Heat the oil in a shallow pan and quickly fry the chicken and onion until golden brown. Add the peppers and cook for 2 – 3 minutes, then stir in the tomatoes, parsley and ground black pepper. Cover tightly and simmer for about 15 minutes until the chicken and vegetables are tender.

SWEET AND SOUR CHICKEN
4 chicken portions (boneless), chopped into smallish pieces
salt
2 tbsp soy sauce (gluten-free)
3 tbsp sunflower oil
1 inch root ginger
1 onion, sliced thinly
1 green pepper, sliced thinly
2 tbsp white wine vinegar
7 oz tin pineapple chunks in its own juice (drained)
1 orange, segmented (optional)
2 tbsp tomato purée
1 tsp cornflour

Heat 2 tablespoons sunflower oil and cook the chicken thoroughly on a medium heat. Remove the chicken and add the ginger, onion and pepper. Cook until soft. Add the vinegar and soy sauce. Mix together. Add the pineapple, orange segments and tomato purée. Dissolve the cornflour in the pineapple juice if you feel it requires thickening. Heat and finally add the chicken. Heat and serve.

CHICKEN IN RED WINE VINEGAR
6 chicken portions or breasts, skin removed
sunflower oil or margarine
6 ripe tomatoes, skinned and chopped
10 fl. oz red wine vinegar
10 fl. oz chicken stock
2 heaped tbsp chopped flat-leaf parsley
salt and pepper

Season the joints of chicken with salt and pepper. Heat 2 oz sunflower oil or margarine in a flameproof casserole until just turning nut brown. Add the chicken and fry gently, turning occasionally until golden brown all over. Add the chopped tomatoes and carry on frying and simmering until the tomato has lost its moisture and is dark red and sticky. Pour in the vinegar and reduce by simmering until almost disappeared. Add the stock and simmer again until reduced by half.

Remove the chicken to a serving dish and keep warm. Whisk the remaining margarine into the sauce to give it a glossy finish. Add 1 tablespoon chopped parsley, pour over the chicken and sprinkle with the remaining parsley.

Meat Dishes

LAMB STEAKS AND CRUNCHY RÖSTI
4 lamb steaks
2 tsp Dijon mustard
2 cloves garlic, peeled and crushed
salt and freshly ground black pepper
4 tbsp oil
1 glass red wine
¼ pint lamb stock
sprigs of flat-leaf parsley for garnish
For the Rösti
2 large waxy potatoes, peeled
½ onion, peeled and finely chopped
1 egg, beaten
1 tbsp finely chopped fresh parsley

Spread steaks with mustard and garlic and season with black pepper. Leave for 20 minutes.

Grate peeled potatoes and put into a bowl, add onion. Add beaten egg, then chopped parsley and seasoning. Heat half the oil in a pan and fry dessertspoonfuls of potato and onion mix until browned on both sides and cooked through. Remove from pan and keep warm. Heat remaining oil in pan and cook lamb steaks to preference. Remove from pan. Reserve and keep warm.

Add wine and stock to pan. Bring to the boil, then simmer until reduced by half. Season. Arrange lamb steaks on rösti, pour over juice and garnish with sprigs of flat-leaf parsley.

BRAISED LAMB WITH CELERY AND LEEKS
4 tbsp oil
2 lb fillet end of leg of lamb
1 onion, peeled and finely chopped
2 leeks, washed, trimmed and chopped
1 head celery, trimmed and chopped
1 pint lamb stock
1 glass white wine
1 tbsp finely chopped fresh parsley
salt and freshly ground black pepper

Heat 2 tablespoons of oil in a pan, and seal and brown lamb on all sides. Lift out with a slotted spoon and place in a flameproof casserole with a tight-fitting lid. Add onion to frying pan with remaining oil and cook gently to soften. Add leeks and celery and cook for a further minute. Transfer to casserole.

Pour over stock and wine. Bring to the boil, then cover. Turn down heat and simmer for 1½ hours or until lamb is tender. Stir in parsley and season with salt and freshly ground black pepper.

MOROCCAN LAMB WITH CHICK-PEAS
1 leg lamb, prepared for roasting
For the Baste
3 tbsp oil
1 tbsp cumin
1 tbsp ground ginger
1 tbsp ground cinnamon
2 cloves garlic, peeled and crushed
good squeeze lemon juice
salt and freshly ground black pepper
2 cloves garlic, peeled and finely crushed
1 onion, peeled and finely chopped
2 tbsp oil
2 x 14 oz (400g) tins chick-peas, drained
Preheat oven to 180°C/350°F/Gas mark 4.

First make the baste. Mix oil with ground cumin, ginger and cinnamon. Stir in garlic and lemon juice. Brush all over the lamb. Season with salt and pepper. Sit on a trivet in a roasting tray. Roast in a preheated oven for 20 minutes per pound, plus 20 minutes. Keep basting throughout cooking. Meanwhile, fry garlic and onion in oil until softened, but not browned. Stir in chick-peas and season. Remove roasting tray from oven 15 minutes before end of cooking time. Lift out lamb on the trivet and add chick-pea mix to roasting tray. Stir to coat in meat juices. Replace lamb and return to oven to finish cooking.

Serve lamb on a platter surrounded by chick-pea mix.

GRILLED LAMB CUTLETS ON ROCKET MASH
This is based on the Irish dish of mashed potatoes with cabbage, called colcannon. Because cooked rocket is very strongly flavoured, you will need only a little for this recipe.
6 lamb cutlets or chops
1 clove garlic
juice of ½ lemon
½ tbsp fresh or dried rosemary
1 tbsp oil
salt and freshly ground pepper

For the Mash
2 lb. floury potatoes
¾ oz rocket
5 tbsp goats' milk or other milk
1½ oz sunflower margarine

Put the lamb chops or cutlets in a bowl. Mix together the next 5 ingredients and pour over the chops. Mix well to coat with the marinade. Leave at room temperature for about an hour, then grill, barbecue or cook in a ridged frying pan until done to your liking.

Meanwhile, peel the potatoes, cut into even-sized pieces and boil in salted water until tender. While the potatoes are cooking, roughly chop the rocket leaves and finely chop any stems. Drain potatoes well, then return to pan and place over a gentle heat for 1–2 minutes, shaking the pan to evaporate leftover water and begin to break up the potatoes. Mash thoroughly, then add salt and pepper to taste. Add sunflower margarine and whisk until margarine is melted. Then whisk in the milk, followed by the rocket.

Oriental Section

ORIENTAL CHICKEN STIR FRY
3 oz skinned and boned chicken breast
½ tsp sesame oil
1 oz red pepper, thinly sliced
1 oz green pepper, thinly sliced
2 oz onion, thinly sliced
2 oz carrot, cut into matchstick lengths
2 oz mushrooms, thinly sliced
3 oz bean sprouts
1 tsp cornflour
2 tsp gluten-free light soy sauce
6 tbsp chicken stock
salt and freshly ground black pepper

Cut the chicken into fine strips.

Heat the oil in a non-stick frying pan and sauté the chicken strips for 3 minutes. Add the peppers, onion and carrot and fry for a further 5 minutes, stirring occasionally. Add mushrooms and cook for 2 minutes. Add the bean sprouts and cook for 1 minute.

Blend cornflour with soy sauce and chicken stock. Add to the pan, stir until boiling, cover and cook for 2 minutes. Season to taste.

FRUITY CURRIED CHICKEN SALAD
2 oz cooked chicken, skin removed
2 oz cooked brown rice
1 oz red pepper, thinly sliced
2 oz halved grapes
3 oz eating apple, cored and diced
1 oz banana, sliced (about half a small banana)
1 tbsp lemon juice
3 tbsp low fat natural yoghurt
salt and pepper
¼ tsp curry powder

Cut the chicken into slivers or small cubes. Put in a bowl with
the rice, pepper slices and grapes. Toss the apple and banana in
the lemon juice, then add to the rice.

Mix the yoghurt with the curry powder, and add salt and
pepper to taste. Lightly fold dressing through the salad.

VEGETABLE CURRY WITH RICE
½ tsp sunflower oil
1 oz onion, finely chopped
1 oz carrot, finely chopped
2 oz cooking apple, cored and chopped
1 tsp curry powder
1 tsp cornflour for thickening
7½ oz tin chopped tomatoes
¼ tsp yeast extract
1 oz chopped leek
2 oz sliced courgette
2 oz cauliflower florets
2 oz French or runner beans, sliced
salt and freshly ground black pepper

Heat the oil in small saucepan and lightly fry the onion, carrot
and apple for about 5 minutes, stirring occasionally. Add the
curry powder and flour and cook gently for 1 minute. Add the

tomatoes, yeast extract and 4 tablespoons water. Bring to the boil, stirring. Add the leek, cover the pan and simmer gently for 15 minutes. Add the remaining vegetables and continue to cook in covered pan for about 10 minutes until all are just tender. Adjust seasoning.

Serve with rice.

SWEET AND SOUR QUORN AND VEGETABLE STIR FRY
14 oz packet Quorn pieces
6 tbsp fresh orange juice
2 tbsp dry sherry
1 tbsp gluten-free dark soy sauce
4 tbsp wine vinegar
1 clove garlic, sliced
1 lb mixed vegetables (e.g. carrots, courgettes, red pepper, mangetout)
3 oz tin water chestnuts, drained
2 tbsp sunflower oil
4 fl. oz vegetable stock
1 tbsp clear honey
1½ level tsp cornflour
4 oz blanched asparagus tips (optional)
salt and freshly ground black pepper

Place the Quorn in a shallow dish. Whisk together the orange juice, sherry, soy sauce and wine vinegar, then add the sliced garlic and pour over the Quorn pieces. Cover and marinate for 1 hour. Strain, reserving the marinade.

Slice the carrots and courgettes. Cut the red pepper into matchsticks, trim the mangetout and slice the water chestnuts.

Heat 1 tablespoon of the oil in a wok or large frying pan. Add the Quorn and stir-fry for 5 minutes or until golden. Remove with a slotted spoon and set aside. Add the remaining oil and fry all the mixed vegetables for 4–5 minutes or until tender. Return the Quorn to the pan with the water chestnuts. Mix the reserved marinade with the vegetable stock, honey and cornflour and stir into the vegetables. Add asparagus tips if using. Cover the pan and simmer for 2–3 minutes.

Season and serve at once.

STIR-FRIED RICE AND QUORN

8 oz rice
8 spring onions
5 carrots
1-inch piece fresh root ginger
14 oz packet Quorn pieces
1 level tsp salt
1 level tsp raw cane sugar
4 tbsp gluten-free soy sauce
2 tbsp dry sherry
3 tbsp sunflower oil
2 x size 2 eggs, lightly beaten

Cook the rice, then drain and set aside to cool. Thinly slice the spring onions. Peel and thinly slice the carrots. Peel and finely shred the ginger.

Mix together the salt, sugar, soy sauce and sherry. Add the Quorn and marinate for 30 minutes.

Heat the oil in a wok or very large frying pan. Add the spring onions, carrot and ginger and stir-fry for 3–4 minutes. Add the Quorn and cook for a further 3 minutes.

Stir in the egg and rice and cook for about 2–3 minutes, until the egg begins to set.

CHILLI WITH RICE

1 lb lean minced beef
1 onion, chopped
1 green pepper, chopped
7½ oz tin chopped tomatoes
15 oz tin red kidney beans (not drained)
14 oz tin tomatoes (not drained)

¼ pint water
1 tbsp chilli powder
1 clove garlic
1 tsp salt
1 bay leaf

In a large saucepan, cook minced beef, onion and green pepper until meat is browned, stirring frequently (pour off surface fat). Stir in remaining ingredients. Cover and cook over low heat for about 1 hour. Stir occasionally.

Serve with boiled rice.

SPICY CHICKEN IN YOGHURT
4 skinned and boned chicken breasts
1 small clove garlic
1 tsp ground coriander
1 tsp ground cumin
½ tsp ground ginger
pinch chilli powder
8 tbsp low fat natural yoghurt

To Serve
brown or white rice
broccoli
carrots, sliced

Make several slashes in the chicken breasts and place in a small dish. Mix garlic and spices with the yoghurt and spread over the chicken. Cover and leave to marinate in refrigerator for 3–4 hours or overnight, turning chicken once.

Remove chicken breasts from marinade and place on a piece of foil in a grill pan. Cook under a medium grill, turning once and brushing with marinade, for about 20 minutes or until the chicken is cooked and golden.

Serve with boiled rice, broccoli and carrots.

MUSHROOM AND LENTIL MOUSSAKA
1¼ lb aubergines, trimmed and thinly sliced
2½ level tsp salt
4 tbsp olive oil
1 large onion, peeled and chopped
1 green pepper, deseeded and chopped
2 cloves garlic, peeled and crushed
8 oz mushrooms, wiped and sliced
12 oz tomatoes, skinned, deseeded and chopped
2 level tsp raw cane sugar
1 level tsp ground cinnamon
freshly ground black pepper
3 tbsp chopped fresh parsley
2 tbsp dry white wine or water
8 oz cooked lentils, drained
1 oz sunflower margarine
1 oz cornflour for thickening
½ pint skimmed milk
2 eggs, separated
¼ level tsp freshly grated or ground nutmeg
4 oz low fat cheese, grated
Preheat oven to 180°C/350°F/Gas mark 4.

Sprinkle the aubergine slices with 2 level teaspoons of the salt and leave for 1 hour. Rinse the slices and pat them dry with kitchen paper.

Heat 2 tablespoons of the oil in a large frying pan and fry the aubergine slices in it until lightly browned on both sides. Put them on a plate and set aside.

Heat the remaining oil in the pan and cook the onion, green pepper and garlic in it for 5 minutes. Stir in the mushrooms, tomatoes, sugar, cinnamon, ¼ teaspoon of the salt, some pepper and the parsley, then pour in the wine or the water. Cover and simmer for 10 minutes. Stir in the lentils, then remove from the heat.

Arrange half the aubergine slices in the bottom of a large ovenproof dish. Spread the lentil mixture evenly over the top, cover with the remaining aubergine slices, then set aside.

Melt the margarine in a saucepan, mix in the cornflour and cook, stirring for 1 minute. Take the pan off the heat and gradually blend in the milk. Return it to the heat and bring to the boil. Cook, stirring for 3–5 minutes or until the sauce thickens.

Remove the pan from the heat and beat in the egg yolks. Season the sauce with the remaining salt, some pepper and the nutmeg. Whisk the egg whites until they hold soft peaks. Mix a quarter of the whites into the sauce, then gently fold in the rest.

Pour the sauce over the aubergines and sprinkle with the cheese. Place in the centre of the oven and bake for 30 minutes.

Turn off the oven and leave the moussaka to settle for 10 minutes before serving.

Garnish with the parsley and serve with a crisp lettuce salad.

CHINESE BEEF AND VEGETABLE STIR FRY
12 oz fillet or rump steak, sliced into very thin strips
2 tbsp cornflour
3 tbsp gluten-free soy sauce
6 tbsp dry sherry
2 tbsp raw cane sugar
2 tbsp red wine vinegar
4 tbsp sesame or vegetable oil
1 onion, thinly sliced
1 clove garlic, crushed
1-inch piece fresh root ginger, peeled and finely chopped
2 sticks celery, thinly sliced
1 red pepper, deseeded and sliced into thin strips
8 oz mangetout, halved

Put steak in a bowl. Mix together the cornflour, soy sauce, sherry, sugar and vinegar, then season to taste. Pour over steak, stir well to coat meat, then cover and leave to marinate for 1 hour.

Heat 2 tablespoons of oil in a wok or large frying pan. Add

onion, garlic and ginger and fry gently, stirring continuously for 5 minutes until soft. Heat another tablespoon of oil in the pan or wok. Add the celery and red pepper and fry, stirring for about a further 5 minutes or until tender but still crisp. Remove vegetables from wok with a slotted spoon and set aside.

Drain steak from marinade. Heat remaining oil in wok, add steak and stir-fry over a high heat for 5 minutes. Remove with a slotted spoon and set aside.

Add the mangetout to the wok and stir-fry for 2–3 minutes. Return steak and vegetables to wok, then pour over the marinade and stir until bubbling and well mixed. Taste and adjust seasoning. Serve at once.

VEGETARIAN PIZZA
4 oz Juvela gluten-free mix
¼ tsp baking powder (see 'My Useful List')
¼ tsp dried mixed herbs
1 oz sunflower margarine
goats' milk or other milk to mix
1 small onion, chopped
1–2 oz mushrooms
2 aubergines
oregano
1 clove garlic (to taste)
14 oz tin tomatoes
Italian seasoning (to taste)
Preheat oven to 200°C/400°F/Gas mark 6.

To make the base, mix together the gluten-free mix, baking powder and mixed herbs. Rub in margarine, then stir in milk to form a soft dough. Knead the dough on a surface dusted with gluten-free mix until smooth. Then roll out or knead onto a pizza dish or baking tray.

To make topping, heat oil in a pan and fry onion until soft and golden. Fry mushrooms, aubergines and garlic. Pour in the tin of tomatoes and add some Italian seasoning and oregano to

taste. Simmer for 10 minutes. Spoon over the base and bake for
25–30 minutes.

QUORN BOLOGNESE
2 tbsp olive oil
1 large onion, chopped
2 cloves garlic, crushed
12 oz minced Quorn
1 tsp dried mixed herbs
Italian seasoning and oregano to taste
red pesto
2 tbsp tomato purée
14 oz tin chopped tomatoes
¼ pint red wine
2 tsp natural cane sugar
salt and freshly ground black pepper
gluten-free pasta to serve

Heat the oil and fry the onion and garlic for 1 minute. Add the
Quorn and dried herbs and fry for 3 minutes. Add red pesto,
tomato purée and chopped tomatoes and stir through. Add wine
and sugar, bring to the boil and simmer for 20 minutes. Season
to taste.
    Serve with gluten-free pasta.

QUORN CHILLI STIR FRY
3 x 15 ml spoons vegetable oil
3 cloves garlic, peeled and crushed
1 inch root ginger, peeled and grated
½ red and ½ green pepper, deseeded and chopped
12 oz (350g) Quorn pieces
6 spring onions, sliced
½ red chilli, thinly sliced (optional)
2 tbsp dry sherry
2 tbsp gluten-free dark soy sauce, if required

1 tbsp white wine vinegar
1 tbsp chilli sauce
1 tbsp natural cane sugar
1 tbsp cornflour
7 fl. oz vegetable stock

Heat oil in a wok or large frying pan and fry garlic, ginger and peppers. Add Quorn, onions and chilli and stir-fry for 4–5 minutes. Stir in sherry until it stops sizzling. Mix remaining ingredients, add to pan and stir-fry for 3 minutes until sauce thickens.

QUORN CHILLI
1 tbsp olive oil
1 small onion
6 oz minced Quorn
1 tsp chilli powder
7½ oz tin chopped tomatoes
¼ pint vegetable stock
½ tbsp Worcestershire sauce
1 tbsp tomato purée
8 oz kidney beans
salt and pepper

Heat the oil in a pan and gently fry the onion and Quorn until the onion is soft. Add the chilli powder and fry for 1 minute. Add the tomatoes, stock, Worcestershire sauce, tomato purée and kidney beans to the pan and mix well. Bring to the boil, cover and simmer gently for 20 minutes. Season to taste.

Serve with rice.

Fish Dishes

FISH AND VEGETABLE GRATIN
4 oz potato, scrubbed
2 oz carrot, sliced
2 oz leek, sliced
2 oz celery, sliced
4 oz white fish, skinned (or smoked fish if preferred)
1 oz shelled prawns
2 tsp cornflour
4 tbsp skimmed milk
pinch grated lemon rind
½ tsp lemon juice
salt and pepper
½ oz grated Cheddar cheese (half fat)

Cut potato into ¼ inch slices, cook in simmering water for 5 minutes, then drain. Meanwhile, put carrot, leek and celery in a small pan, just cover with water and simmer for 5 minutes. Arrange fish on top of vegetables and continue simmering until fish is just cooked (about 10 minutes).

Remove fish and vegetables from pan. Remove any bones from fish, divide into large flakes and arrange with vegetables and prawns in an ovenproof dish.

Measure reserved fish stock in pan, making up to ¼ pint (150 ml) with cold water, if necessary. Blend cornflour with milk and add to fish stock. Bring to the boil, stirring. Add lemon rind, juice and seasoning to taste. Pour over fish and vegetables.

Arrange sliced potato over the top, sprinkle with cheese. Cook under a moderate grill or in the oven at 190ºC/375ºF/Gas mark 5, for about 10–15 minutes, until golden.

FISH PROVENÇALE
½ tsp sunflower oil
1 oz finely chopped onion
1 oz finely chopped celery
small clove garlic, crushed
7½ oz tin chopped tomatoes
2 tsp tomato purée
1 tsp chopped fresh basil (optional)
salt and pepper
4 oz boned and skinned white fish

Heat the oil in a small saucepan, add the onion, celery and garlic and cook gently for 5 minutes. Add the tinned and puréed tomatoes, basil and seasoning. Bring to the boil and simmer for 15–20 minutes, stirring occasionally, until the sauce is well cooked and thickened.

Cut fish into large cubes. Add to the pan, cover and simmer for a further 10 minutes.

Adjust seasoning.

Serve with cooked rice or gluten-free pasta and green salad, garnished with basil.

GOLDEN TOPPED PLAICE (SERVES 1)
For each Plaice Fillet:
1 oz celery, finely chopped
2 oz apple, cored and grated
pinch grated lemon rind
2 tsp lemon juice
2 tsp chopped fresh parsley
½ oz gluten-free breadcrumbs
salt and pepper

plaice fillet
half fat Cheddar cheese (optional amount to taste)

Put celery, apple, lemon rind and 1 teaspoon (5 ml) lemon juice
in a small pan with 1 tablespoon water. Cover and cook gently
until celery is just softened. Remove lid and continue to cook
until liquid has evaporated (about 2 minutes), stirring
occasionally. Add chopped parsley, breadcrumbs and seasoning
to taste. Place fish, skin side down, on a piece of foil and sprinkle
over remaining lemon juice. Grill under a moderate grill for
about 5 minutes. Spoon topping over fish and cook for a further
3 minutes. Sprinkle with cheese and continue to grill for 2–3
minutes or until cheese has melted.

Cakes and Breads

Cakes

JAYNE'S TEA LOAF
12 oz mixed dried fruit
10 fl. oz cold tea
6 oz natural raw cane sugar
1 large egg
9 oz brown rice flour
3 oz ground almonds
1 oz chopped almonds
Preheat oven to 180°C/350°F/Gas mark 4.
Two 1 lb loaf tins, greased and lined

Put the fruit into a bowl and pour over the cold tea. Leave for 4 hours or overnight. Beat sugar and egg, then mix in fruit and tea mixture. Fold in flour, ground almonds and chopped almonds. Divide mixture into the two loaf tins. Put the tins in the centre of the oven for 1 hour. Cool on a wire tray. Store for 24 hours before use.

This is nice sliced and buttered or eaten as a cake.

Suitable for freezing.

EASY FRUIT CAKE
22 oz mixed dried fruit
2 oz flaked almonds

6 oz raw cane sugar
4 oz sunflower margarine
1 tsp mixed spice
2 eggs
½ tsp bicarbonate of soda
½ pint goats' milk
12 oz brown rice flour (or 10 oz brown rice flour with 2 oz
    ground almonds)
Preheat oven to 190°C/375°F/Gas mark 5.
9-inch-deep cake tin, greased and lined

Put the fruit and nuts, sugar, margarine, spice, bicarbonate of
soda and milk into a large bowl. Microwave on high for 10
minutes, stirring frequently. Cool. Stir in the flour and eggs. Mix
well. Spoon the mixture into a prepared tin and slightly hollow
out the centre.

Put the tin in the centre of the oven and cook for 1¼ hours.

SEMI-RICH FRUIT CAKE
5 oz sunflower margarine
5 oz raw cane sugar
2 eggs
11 oz (275g) mixed fruit
4–5 tbsp goats' milk
5 oz brown rice flour, sieved together with 1 tsp mixed spice
3 oz ground almonds
Preheat oven to 150°C/300°F/Gas mark 2.
7-inch cake tin, greased

Mix margarine and sugar until light and fluffy. Add the eggs one
at a time. Add the sieved flour, ground almonds and milk. Add
the fruit and mix again.

Bake in a preheated oven for approximately 2 hours, until
cooked.

DATE AND RICE CRISPIE SLICE
5 oz sunflower margarine
1 cup raw cane sugar
pinch salt
1 cup chopped dates
1 tsp vanilla essence
4 cups Rice Krispies

Grease a tray measuring 8 x 12 inches.

Place margarine, sugar, salt, dates and vanilla in saucepan. Simmer on low heat for 5 minutes. Gently stir in Rice Crispies. Spread on greased tray and place in fridge until set.

Cut into squares when cold.

APPLE SPONGE
Stewed Apples
6–8 cooking apples
½ cup raw cane sugar
4–8 tbsp water
4 cloves

Peel, core and slice apples. Place all ingredients in a saucepan and simmer gently until the apples are tender. Place in a greased casserole.

Sponge Topping
1¼ cups rice flour
½ cup soya flour
3 tsp baking powder
½ cup raw cane sugar
5 oz sunflower margarine
⅔ cup milk
2 eggs
1 tsp vanilla essence
Preheat oven to 175ºC/350ºF/Gas mark 4.

Combine all ingredients. Beat for 3 minutes in a mixer. Pour mixture over stewed apples and bake for 50–60 minutes.

STICKY CHOCOLATE CAKE
3 oz sunflower margarine
9 oz dark muscovado sugar
5 tbsp cocoa powder
3 eggs
4 oz ground rice or rice flour
3 oz ground almonds
1 tsp gluten-free baking powder
Preheat oven to 180°C/350°F/Gas mark 4.

Line an 8-inch (20 cm) square cake tin with greaseproof paper.
Beat together fat and sugar until light and fluffy. Bring 3½ fl. oz (100 ml) water to the boil, then whisk in the cocoa powder until well blended. Fold blended cocoa into the creamed mixture.
Beat in the eggs one at a time and add 1 tablespoon of ground rice or rice flour with each addition. Fold in remaining ground rice or flour, ground almonds and baking powder. Turn the mixture into the tin and smooth the top. Bake for 35 minutes until firm. Cool on a wire rack, then cut into squares.

BASIC SPONGE MIX
½ oz soya flour
1 oz raw cane sugar
½ level tsp dried pectin
¾ oz potato flour
2 oz ground brown rice
½ oz yellow split pea flour
½ oz ground almonds
1 tbsp gluten-free baking powder (slightly heaped)
5 tbsp orange juice
2 tbsp sunflower oil

Preheat oven to 200ºC/400ºF/Gas mark 6.

Put all ingredients into a bowl and mix with a wooden spoon until you have a creamy cake mix.

Divide into 6 bun tins.

Bake on the top shelf for about 15 minutes, until golden.

Cool on a wire rack and eat on the day they are made.

BIRTHDAY CAKE

2 oz soya flour

3 oz raw cane sugar

2 tsp dried pectin

6 oz ground brown rice

1 oz yellow split pea flour

4 oz ground almonds

1 tbsp gluten-free baking powder (slightly heaped)

2 heaped tsp gluten-free spice

1 heaped tsp cinnamon

3 tbsp sunflower oil

⅔ pint pure orange juice

6 oz finely grated eating apple

2 oz finely grated carrot

rind of 1 lemon and 1 orange, coarsely grated

1 lb dried mixed fruit

Preheat oven to 200ºC/400ºF/Gas mark 6.

8-inch round cake tin, oiled and floured with ground brown rice

Put the first 9 ingredients into a bowl and mix well. Add the oil, orange juice, grated apple and carrot. Mix again. Stir in the rinds and the fruit.

Spoon the cake mixture into the tin and flatten the top with a knife.

Bake near the top of the oven for about 1 hour.

Leave for a minute or two before turning out on to a wire rack to cool.

Store in an airtight container and use within 7 to 8 days.

MADEIRA CAKE
1 oz soya flour
2 oz raw cane sugar
1 tsp dried pectin
1½ oz potato flour
4 oz ground brown rice
¾ oz yellow split pea flour
1 oz ground almonds
1 tsp gluten-free baking powder (slightly heaped)
juice of a fresh lemon, made up to ½ pint with water
3 oz finely grated apple
2 tbsp vegetable oil
grated rind of 1 lemon
Preheat oven at 200°C/400°F/Gas mark 6.
Loaf tin measuring 7¼ x 3½ x 2¼ inches, oiled and floured with
    ground brown rice

Put all ingredients into a bowl and mix with a wooden spoon
until you have a creamy cake mix.

Spoon the mixture into the loaf tin. Flatten the top with a
knife and bake on the top shelf for about 40 minutes. Turn out
on to a wire rack to cool.

BREAD AND BUTTER PUDDING
6–8 slices bread (crusts removed) (gluten-free if possible)
2 oz sunflower margarine
2 oz sultanas
grated rind of lemon (optional)
2 eggs
¾ pint goats' milk or soya milk
3 tbsp raw cane sugar
pinch grated nutmeg
Preheat oven to 180°C/350°F/Gas mark 4.

Thickly spread the slices of bread with margarine and cut into
triangles. Place half in an ovenproof dish. Sprinkle over half the

sultanas, half the lemon rind and top with the remaining bread, buttered side uppermost.

Beat together the eggs, milk, sugar and nutmeg and pour over the bread. Sprinkle over the remaining lemon and sultanas.

Allow to stand for 15 minutes, then bake in preheated oven for 1 hour until crispy and golden.

GERMAN APPLE CAKE
2 oz sunflower margarine
⅓ cup raw cane sugar
1 egg
⅔ cup rice flour
⅓ cup soya flour
2 tsp baking powder
¼ cup milk (goats' milk/soya milk optional)
3 medium apples
juice of 1 lemon
cinnamon and extra sugar
½ tsp vanilla essence
Preheat oven to 175ºC/350ºF/Gas mark 4.
One 8-inch round cake tin, greased

Cream margarine and sugar in a large bowl or mixer. Add egg and beat well. Sift flours and baking powder. Add half flour mixture to egg mixture and beat. Add milk and remaining flour alternately. Spread over base of tin.

Peel, quarter and remove core from apples. Cut into thin slices and squeeze lemon juice over. Arrange slices over cake mixture. Bake for approximately 1 hour. Sprinkle with extra sugar and cinnamon.

CARROT CAKE
1½ cups rice flour
1 cup raw cane sugar
½ tsp salt

1 tsp bicarbonate of soda
½ cup crushed pineapple (undrained)
1 cup grated carrot
2 eggs
½ cup oil
½ tsp vanilla essence
½ cup chopped walnuts
Preheat oven to 175ºF/350ºC/Gas mark 4.
Loaf tin measuring 8 x 4 inches, lined

Sift flour, sugar, salt and bicarbonate of soda into a large bowl.
Add pineapple, carrot, eggs, oil and vanilla. Beat until combined,
then stir in the nuts.

Pour into the prepared loaf tin and bake for 60–70 minutes.

SPICED CURRANT COOKIES
2 oz sunflower margarine
4 oz ground brown rice
3 oz finely grated eating apple
1½ oz raw cane sugar
½ tsp mixed spice
1½ oz currants
Preheat oven to 230ºC/450ºF/Gas mark 8.
Baking sheet, greased

In a bowl, blend the margarine and ground rice with a fork. Add
the apple, sugar, spice and currants. Knead and mix with a
wooden spoon until a ball of dough is formed.

Put 8–10 spoonfuls of the dough on to the greased baking
sheet. Spread out into cookie shapes with a knife. Bake for about
20–25 minutes.

Allow the cookies to cool on baking sheet.

MACAROONS
6 oz ground almonds
6 oz caster sugar (raw cane sugar), plus extra for sprinkling
2–3 drops vanilla essence
2 egg whites
a few blanched almonds for decoration
Preheat oven to 180ºC/350ºF/Gas mark 4.
Line 2 large baking trays with non-stick baking parchment

Mix ground almonds and sugar together in a mixing bowl, then stir in vanilla essence. Lightly beat egg whites, then gradually stir into almond mixture, adding enough to give a fairly stiff consistency – the mixture should be firm enough to hold its shape.

Place heaped tablespoonfuls of the mixture on to the baking trays, spacing well apart to allow for spreading. Place an almond in the centre of each and sprinkle lightly with caster sugar.

Bake for about 15 minutes until firm and lightly coloured. Leave to cool on trays for 2 minutes, then transfer to wire racks to finish cooling.

CHRISTMAS PUDDING
1 oz plain gluten-free flour
⅛ tsp salt
¼ tsp gluten-free mixed spice
⅛ tsp bicarbonate of soda
grated rind of ½ lemon
2 oz cooking apple, grated
2 oz brown sugar
1 oz chopped almonds
2 oz sultanas
2 oz currants
1 oz raisins
3–4 tbsp goats' or soya milk
1½ oz gluten-free shredded suet
2½ oz gluten-free breadcrumbs

1 medium-sized egg
1 lb pudding basin, greased

Stir the flour, salt, mixed spice and bicarbonate of soda into a large mixing bowl. Add the lemon rind, apple, sugar, almonds, dried fruit, shredded suet and breadcrumbs. Mix well. Beat the egg with the milk. Gradually stir into the mixture, which should form a soft dropping consistency. If it is too stiff, add a little more milk. Spoon into the basin, cover with greased greaseproof paper and then with foil. Place in a steamer or in a covered pan containing water halfway up the sides of the basin. Bring to the boil and steam for 5 hours, topping up with boiling water as necessary. Allow to cool. Cover with new foil or a cloth and seal well.

When ready to use, steam for 1–1½ hours and serve.

This pudding improves with keeping and can be stored for up to a year. If it becomes dry, moisten with a little cider or milk before resteaming.

TEACUP CAKE
1 teacup cold tea (without milk)
1 teacup unrefined sugar
1 teacup mixed dried fruit
2 oz sunflower margarine
1 large egg
sieve together: 1 teacup soya flour
                    1 teacup brown rice flour
                    2 tsp baking powder
¼ teacup chopped almonds or walnuts (optional)
Preheat oven to 180ºC/350ºF/Gas mark 4.
2 lb loaf tin, greased and lined

In a saucepan, put the tea, sugar, margarine and fruit. Bring to simmering point and simmer for 2–3 minutes. Take the pan off the heat and allow to cool until lukewarm.

Add the beaten egg and sieved flour. Mix all together with a wooden spoon and finally add the nuts. Pour into the prepared loaf tin and bake for 1–1¼ hours.

CHRISTMAS CAKE
5 oz sunflower margarine
5 oz soft brown sugar
8 oz plain gluten-free flour
½ tsp gluten-free baking powder
1 tsp gluten-free mixed spice
3 medium-sized eggs
15 oz mixed dried fruit
2 oz ground almonds
2–4 tbsp goats' or soya milk
Preheat oven to 170°C/325°F/Gas mark 3.
Grease a 7-inch square cake tin or an 8-inch round cake tin and
    line with two layers of greaseproof paper.

Cream the margarine and sugar until soft. Sift together the flour, baking powder and mixed spice. Beat in the eggs one at a time with a teaspoonful of flour, beating well each time. Fold in half the sifted flour. Then fold in the dried fruit, together with the rest of the flour and the ground almonds. The mixture should be of a heavy dropping consistency. If it is too stiff, add 2–4 tablespoonfuls of milk. Spoon into the prepared tin and bake for 1½ hours in the middle of the oven. Then lower the oven temperature to 150°C/300°F/Gas mark 2, cover the top with two sheets of greaseproof paper and cook for a further 1–1½ hours until a skewer comes out clean. Cool on a wire rack and, when cold, wrap with its greaseproof paper, in foil.
    Allow to mature for several days.
    Cover with gluten-free marzipan if desired.

BREAD
2 slightly heaped tsp dried yeast granules (if fresh yeast is used, double the amount)
9 fl. oz warm water
1 heaped tsp raw cane sugar
1 oz soya flour
4½ oz potato flour
¾ oz yellow split pea flour
¾ oz ground almonds
2 pinches sea salt
2 tsp vegetable or sunflower oil
Preheat oven to 180°C/350°F/Gas mark 4.
Loaf tin measuring 7¼ x 3½ x 2¼ inches, oiled and floured

Sprinkle the yeast into warm water with the sugar and leave.

Put all the other ingredients into a bowl and mix well.

Stir the yeast, water and sugar together and pour onto the flour mixture. Mix, then beat to a creamy consistency with a wooden spoon. Do not use a mixer.

Put mixture into prepared tin and bake for 1 hour.

FRUIT AND PECAN NUT CAKE
3 oz sunflower margarine
2 oz raw cane sugar
2 tbsp marmalade (sugar free)
2 eggs
6 oz potato flour
½ tsp salt
1 tsp gluten-free baking powder
4 oz pecan nuts or walnuts
8 oz raisins or sultanas
Preheat oven to 140°C/275°F/Gas mark 1.
Grease and line a 6-inch round tin or loaf tin.

Cream the margarine and sugar together until pale and light, then beat in the marmalade and eggs.

Sift together the flour, salt and baking powder and fold into the marmalade mixture.

Chop the nuts and add them with the dried fruit to the mixture.

Spoon the mixture into the tin and bake for 1½–2 hours or until a skewer inserted in the centre of the cake comes out clean.

Leave to cool on a wire rack. When cold, wrap in greaseproof paper.

My Useful List

BAKING POWDER   2 parts cream of tartar
                                    1 part bicarbonate of soda

POTATO FLOUR, PEA FLOUR
SOYA FLOUR   For bread
RICE FLOUR   For cakes
GROUND RICE/FLAKED RICE   For puddings
MAIZE FLOUR (CORN MEAL)   For gravy
*Please note: Only use gluten-free products if applicable

PRODUCT	BRAND	MANUFACTURER/SUPPLIER
Fruit and Nut Organic Bars	Shepherdboy Ltd.	Cross Street,
		Syston, Leicester, LE7 2JG.
Gluten-free soy sauce		
Peanut butter		Tyn, Llidiart House
Various fruit spreads	Meridian	Corwen, Clwyd,
Pasta sauce	Foods	LL21 9RJ
Sauces		(tel. 01490-413151)
Mincemeat		
Ice cream dessert	Winner UK Ltd.	Waterside Point 2,
		Anholt Road, London,
		SW11 4PD.
		(tel. 0207-924-6928)
Live fruit yoghurt	Ann Forshaw Yoghurt	Alston Dairy Ltd, Alston
		Lane, Alston, Longridge,
		Preston, Lancashire PR3 3BN
		(tel. 01772-782621)

Gluten-free bread mix	Juvela	SHS International Ltd., 100 Wavertree Boulevard, Wavertree Technology Park, Liverpool, L7 9PT. (tel. 0151-228-1992)
Gluten-free pasta Gluten-free short-cut spaghetti Gluten-free macaroni	Nutricia Dietary Products Ltd.	Newmarket Avenue, White Horse Business Park, Trowbridge, Wiltshire, BA14 0XQ. (tel. 01225-768381)
Just Bouillon stock cubes (no artificial colours or additives) Puffed rice cakes Puffed rice breakfast cereal	Kallo Foods Ltd.	Sunbury-on-Thames, Middlesex, TW16 7JZ.
Bread (fresh) Bread mixes Lasagne (fresh) Pizza bases (fresh) Flour	Ultrapharm Ltd.	Centenary Business Park, Henley-on-Thames, Oxfordshire, RG9 1DF. (tel. 01491-578016)

Things You Can Eat

Provamel Yogu 100 per cent non-dairy yoghurts

Meridian fruit spread

Energi rice loaf – yeast-free, gluten-free, wheat-free, with no added sugar, low in saturates and a good source of fibre, 612g. This is very expensive bread, so maybe if you talk to your doctor nicely, he will give you it on prescription.

Kallo organic dark chocolate rice cakes – these are great as an occasional treat, especially if you miss chocolate.

Plain salted crisps, preferably organic – these make a nice little treat.

Try going into your local health food shop. You will find they have lots of things for you to nibble at! Such as – lightly salted roasted broad beans, luxury dried mango, and a definite treat called Apricot Delight (this is made with apricots, pears, prunes and sugar).

RICE PUDDING (TO MAKE A 2-PINT PUDDING)

1 carton Provamel rice milk – original or vanilla

or

1 carton soya milk – original, vanilla or sweetened

2 oz white pudding rice (use 1 oz white pudding rice per pint of milk)

1 oz fruit sugar (optional)

½ oz soya margarine per 2 pints of milk

Meridian fruit spread (jam)

Preheat oven to hottest setting.

Place all the ingredients into a suitably sized casserole dish. Put it in the centre of the oven and then bring to the boil, stirring every 15 minutes.

When pudding is boiling, reduce the heat to a moderate setting.

Continue to cook the pudding, stirring every 15 minutes. When the pudding reaches a creamy consistency and the rice is soft, the pudding is ready.

Remove from oven. Allow to cool a little before eating. A little sugar-free jam may be added is desired.

This can be eaten cold.

BAKED POTATO
baking potato
soya spread or sunflower spread
garlic salt
extra virgin olive oil, sunflower oil or safflower oil

All you have to do for a baked potato is prick it a few times and put it in the oven for approximately 1–1½ hours at 150ºC/300ºF/Gas mark 2.

To make it interesting, I cover the whole potato with garlic olive oil (which you can make very simply by adding 1–2 chopped cloves of garlic to your olive oil) and sprinkle all over with garlic salt.

After baking, cut open and put soya or sunflower spread on.

Try experimenting by sprinkling chopped chives, tuna fish, etc. on top.

MASHED POTATO
Quite simply, use soya margarine or sunflower margarine instead of butter, and try using a non-dairy milk.

STEAMED VEGETABLES
You can use any vegetables and in any quantity that you like. Simply cut and prepare your vegetables, put them in the steamer and steam until the vegetables are still slightly crunchy.

GRAVY
½ tsp Marmite
½ pint boiling water
3 tsp cornflour per ½ pint of liquid
salt to taste
jelly of a chicken – when you drain the fat off a chicken, leave to cool so that the fat and the jelly separate. Discard the fat and use the jelly

Place the jelly of the chicken and some of the boiling water into a jug. When dissolved, very carefully stir in the cornflour, then stir in some Marmite and salt to taste. Then simply add the rest of the water. Try replacing chicken jelly with beef jelly.

WHITE SAUCE
1 oz cornflour
4 oz non-dairy milk
seasoning to taste

Place the flour and the seasoning in a bowl, mix together, then gradually add milk. When it is all mixed smoothly together, heat up until thickened. To make more of this sauce, just double, treble, etc. the ingredients.

Parsley Sauce: simple add as much parsley to your white sauce as you like.

Non-Dairy Spread Sauce: simply add 1 oz spread to the sauce and mix in.

APPLE CRUMBLE
Stewed Fruit
4 large cooking apples or 1–2 lb fruit of your choice
¾ oz fruit sugar
Crumble
8 oz rice flour
3 oz soya or sunflower margarine
1 oz fruit sugar
Preheat oven to 160°C.

Peel, core and slice the apples into a saucepan with ¾ oz fruit sugar and 4 tablespoons of water. Place on hob and cook gently until soft, stirring frequently. Place cooked apple into a large casserole dish.

Place flour and margarine into a mixing bowl. Rub margarine into flour until it resembles fine breadcrumbs. Stir in 1 oz fruit sugar. Pour crumble mixture over cooked fruit.

Place in centre of preheated oven for approximately 45–50 minutes until golden brown.

Remove from oven and cool for 5 minutes.

CUSTARD (THIS MAKES ¼ PINT CUSTARD)
1 oz rice flour
½ oz fruit sugar
1 egg
¼ pint non-dairy milk
drop of vanilla essence if desired

Mix the flour and sugar together. Beat the egg in a cup and heat the milk. It is at this point you may add the vanilla essence if you want to. I do this in the microwave, but it is equally as successful on the hob. Carefully add the beaten egg to the rice flour and sugar. When you have a smooth paste, gradually add the warmed milk. When this is all mixed in, put back into the microwave and stir every few seconds until at the consistency you like.

GROUND RICE
1 pint non-dairy milk
2 oz ground rice
1 oz fruit sugar

The easiest way to make this is in a microwave, but it can also be made on the hob.

Place the fruit sugar, ground rice and some of the milk into a bowl and mix into a paste. Add the remainder of the milk. Put into a microwave for approximately 5 minutes, stirring every few seconds. You need to do this often, otherwise it will go lumpy. Add a teaspoonful of jam if required.

SMOOTHIE
2 flavoured Provamel yoghurts
any variety and quantity of fresh fruit

Place the yoghurts and fruit (e.g. two kiwis, two peaches, a quarter of a melon, 6–7 strawberries, 3–4 plums and some pineapple) in a blender and mix until smooth. This should make approximately 2 pints, which is enough for 2–3 days. Store in the fridge once made up. This makes a really tasty alternative to breakfast cereals.

TOAST
Energi rice loaf

Toast bread as you would do with normal bread and put soya or sunflower margarine on. Then eat.

Although this looks like normal bread, do not try and make a sandwich with it – it's horrible!

Try this with fruit spread or with Marmite and no margarine.

Also, why not poach a couple of eggs and have this for your breakfast or tea?

FISH PIE
6 pieces of cod fillet
fresh parsley to taste
1 leek
approximately 12 potatoes
1 pint non-dairy milk
4 oz rice flour/cornflour
salt to taste
Preheat oven to 180ºC/250ºF/Gas Mark 4.

Peel the potatoes, add salt to taste, boil and then mash when cooked using non-dairy margarine and non-dairy milk. Using a steamer, steam the cod fillets and, if you have two compartments in your steamer, place the finely chopped leek into the other compartment. While this is cooking, prepare the sauce. I prefer to use the microwave, but it can easily be done on the hob. Put the flour into a dish and gradually add your heated milk. Put this back on to the heat or in the microwave and keep heating gently until this thickens, stirring constantly. When it is thick enough, add the chopped parsley and salt to taste. When the fish fillets and the leek are cooked, flake the fish fillets, add the leeks and pour in the prepared sauce. Mix this well together and pour into a large Pyrex dish. Place the mashed potato on top of the fish mixture and place in the preheated oven for about 30 minutes.

I make this amount so that I can put at least six separate servings into the freezer, as this dish is quite time-consuming to make. It would be very simple to make this in small amounts. For the sauce, the rule of thumb is 1 oz flour to a ¼ pint milk.

Tip! You could quite easily make this into a vegetarian dish. Instead of fish, just add one or two more cooked vegetables, but leave the leek in.

Another Tip! If, like me, you do not use fresh parsley all the time and you find you have to buy a bunch, simply use the amount that you want, then put the rest straight into the freezer and use when needed.

Bibliography and Literature

Dijk, Dr Paul van – *Geneeswijzen.*Uitgeverij Ankh Hermes b.v., Deventer, the Netherlands.

Edelhardt, Mike with Dr Jean Lindeman – *Interferon.* Ballantine Books. Ed. April 1982.

Enzypharm Biochemicals Limited – *A Manual of Enzyme Therapy.* P.O. Box 69, Harrogate, Yorks.

Graham, Judy – *Multiple Sclerosis – A Self-Help Guide to Its Management.* Thorsons Publishers Ltd. 1981.

Horne, Ross – *The Health Revolution* (First Edition 1980). Ross Horne, Avalon Beach, NSW, Australia.

James, Dr P.B. – *Multiple Sclerosis – Many Scars and Hyperbaric Oxygen Therapy.* Wolfson Institute, Dundee University.

MacDougall, Roger – *My Fight Against Multiple Sclerosis.* Regenics Limited. 1975.

Russell Manning, Betsy – *How Safe are Silver/Mercury Fillings?* P.O. Box 691, Catostoga, Cal. 94515, USA. 1983.

'Uw Richtlijn' – *Publications.* Redaktie: Kapellenberglaan 2, Rozendal (Gld.), the Netherlands.

Vogel, A. – *The Nature Doctor* (Eighth Edition 1977). Verlag A. Vogel Teufen/AR/Switzerland.

Index

Acupuncture 63–7, 74
  auriculo 65–6
  electro 65
  restoration 66
Alcohol 62, 74–5
  not permitted 28, 75
  permitted 30
Alexander Technique
  81
Alzheimer's disease 71
Animal fat-free diet 22,
  25, 28, 35
  supplementing 26–7,
  49
Apple Cake, German
  126
Apple Crumble 138
Apple Sponge 122–3
Arachidonic acids 29
ARMS organisation 60
Arsenic 33
Artificial sweeteners 30
Asai, Prof Karl 58
Autism 83

Bathing 32
  cold water 78–9
Beans 31
Beans, soya 31
Beef 30
Beef & Vegetable Stir
  Fry, Chinese
  113–14
Birthday Cake 124
Boericke, Dr William
  70
Bread 131
Bread & Butter

Pudding 125–6
Breathing exercises 62
Buttermilk 30

Cakes
  Birthday Cake 124
  Carrot Cake 126–7
  Christmas Cake 130
  Easy Fruit Cake
  120–1
  Fruit & Pecan Nut
  Cake 131
  German Apple Cake
  126–7
  Jayne's Tea Loaf 120
  Madeira Cake 125
  Semi-Rich Fruit
  Cake 121
  Sticky Chocolate
  Cake 123–4
  Teacup Cake 129–30
Calcium 26, 49
Cannellini Chicken 95
Carob 30
Carrot Cake 126–7
Cereals 28, 29
Cheese 30
Chicken dishes
  Chicken &
  Mushroom
  Fricassee 98–9
  Chicken Casserole
  96–7
  Chicken in Barbecue
  Sauce 97
  Chicken in Red Wine
  Vinegar 101–2
  Chicken Marengo 96

Chicken Risotto 98
Cannellini Chicken
  95
Fruity Curried
  Chicken Salad 108
Harlequin Chicken
  100–1
Indian-Style Chicken
  100
Oriental Stir Fry
  Chicken 107
Spanish-Style Rice
  with Chicken 99
Spicy Chicken in
  Yoghurt 111
Sweet & Sour
  Chicken 101
Chilli, Quorn 116
Chilli Stir Fry, Quorn
  116
Chilli with Rice
  110–11
Chinese Beef &
  Vegetable Stir Fry
  113–14
Chips 29
Chocolate 30
  Chocolate Cake 123
Christmas Cake 130
Christmas Pudding
  128–9
Cod liver oil 51
Coeliac disease 25
Coffee 30
'Cold Dip' 79
Cold water washing
  78–9
Colour therapy 66–7

INDEX

Conversion tables 86–7
Copper 52
Crisps 29
Custard 138

Dairy products 22, 25, 28, 35
Date & Rice Krispie Slice 122
Dental fillings 68–73
Diabetes 25
Dismutase 51

EFA (essential fatty acids) 55–6
Egg & Vegetable Bake 93–4
Eggs 30
Euphoria 79–80
Evening primrose oil 47, 51, 53–7
Evers, Dr Ray 58–60
Exercises 75–82

Fat embolism 60
Fatty acids 29, 55–6
Feta & Mushroom Risotto 92
Fish 30
Fish & Vegetable Gratin 117–18
Fish oils 51, 55
Fish Pie 140
Fish Provencale 118
Folic Acid 27, 49
Forbes, Bryan, *A Divided Life* 41–8, 84
Free-range meat 28, 31
Fresh air, importance of 32
Fresh food, importance of 31–2
Fried food 28
Fruit 29, 49
Fruit, dried 29
Fruit & Pecan Nut Cake 131–2
Fruit Cake, Semi-Rich 121
Fruit Cake, Easy 120–1
Fruit juice 29–30, 32

Germanium 51, 58, 61
GLA (gamma linoleic acid) 53–4
Gluten-free bread 29
Gluten-free diet/food 22, 25, 28, 29, 35, 45, 83, 85
supplementing 26–7, 49
Glycogen 62
Gravy 137
Gregoriades 52

Harlequin Chicken 100–1
Hassam, Dr 55
HBO (Hyperbaric Oxygen treament) 58–9
Honey 30
Hunter-gatherer diet 18, 22–3
Hypoglycaemia 25

Immunoglobins 50
Indian-Style Chicken 100
Ingredients, checking 31
Interferon 50, 51
Iron 52
Issell, Dr 70

James, Dr 60–1
Jayne's Tea Loaf 120

Khoe, Dr Willem 68, 71

Lamb, Braised, with Celery & Leeks 104
Lamb, Moroccan, with Chick-Peas 104–5
Lamb Cutlets, Grilled, on Rocket Mash 105–6
Lamb Steaks & Crunchy Rosti 103
Lecithin 27, 49
Lecitone 52
Legumes 31
Lentil Soup 89
Lentils 31, 112
Linoleic/linoleic acid 29
Lipid complexes 52
Liver 61–2, 75

Lying down exercise 78
Lymphocytes 51, 62

Macaroons 128
MacDougall, Roger 17
Mad cow disease 36–7
Madeira Cake 125
Magnesium 52
Manner, Dr Harold 50
Manning, Betsy Russell, *How Safe are Silver (Mercury) Fillings?* 68–70
Meat, canned 30
Meat eating 28, 30
Melon & Grapefruit Cocktail 88
Mercury toxicity 68–73
Milk 22–3, 36, 28
Mineral supplements 26–7, 35, 45, 49, 51–2
Minestrone 89–90
Moolenburgh, Dr H. 80
Moussaka, Mushroom & Lentil 112–13
Multiple sclerosis description & symptoms of, 21–2
possible genetic basis 36
virus as cause of 50
Mushroom & Feta Risotto 92
Mushroom & Lentil Moussaka 112–13
Myelin sheaths 21, 36, 60

Newman, Nanette 43–4, 46–8
Fun Food Feasts 47
The Fun Food Factory 47
Nuts 30
Nystagmus 24, 32

Offal 30, 31
Olive oil 56
Oriental Stir Fry Chicken 107
Osteopathy 82
Oxygen 58–62

Parkinson's Disease 36
PD capsule 57
Penzer, Dr Victor 73
Phospholipid transfers 52
Pizza, Vegetarian 114–15
Plaice, Gold Topped 118–19
Posture 75–6, 78
Potatoes 31
  baked 136
  mashed 136
Pumpkin seeds 30

Quorn & Rice, Stir Fry 110
Quorn & Vegetable Stir Fry, Sweet & Sour 109–10
Quorn Bolognese 115
Quorn Chilli 116
Quorn Chilli Stir Fry 115–16

Ratatouille, Oven-roasted 91
Raw food 32
Reflexology 82
Relaxation 62
Rice 29, 49–50
  Chilli with Rice 110–11
  Ground Rice 139
  Rice & Quorn Stir Fry 110
  Rice loaf toast 139
  Rice Pudding 135–6
  Rice with Summer Vegetables 92–3
  Spanish-style Rice with Chicken 99
  Vegetable Curry with Rice 109
Risotto, Chicken 98
Risotto, Feta & Mushroom 92

Sago, 30, 31
Salads 29
Saturated fats 26, 27, 54
Schizophrenia 83

Selenium 52
Sitting posture 75–6
  exercises for 76–7
Smoking 62, 74
Smoothie 139
Soups
  Lentil 89
  Minestrone 89–90
  Tomato 90
  Watercress & Potato 88
Soy sauce 85
Spanish-Style Rice with Chicken 99
Spiced Currant Cookies 127
Spicy Chicken in Yoghurt 111
Spinach 31
Sponge mix, basic 123–4
Soya beans, 31
Standing & moving 77, 78
Sticky Chocolate Cake 123
Store cupboard basics 133–4
Sugar, unrefined 28
Sugar-free diet 22, 25, 28, 35
Sunflower oil 55-6
Sunflower seeds 30
Super oxide radical 50, 51
Sweet & Sour Chicken 101
Sweet & Sour Vegetable & Quorn Stir Fry 109–10
Symonds, Sir Charles 20

Tapioca 30, 31
Tea 30
Teacup Cake 129–30
Thomson, Walter 66
Thymosine 51
Toast, rice loaf 139
Tomato Soup 90

Vegetable & Egg Bake 93–4

Vegetable & Fish Gratin 117–18
Vegetable & Quorn Stir Fry, Sweet & Sour 109–10
Vegetable Curry with Rice 108–9
Vegetable juice 29–30, 32
Vegetable Stir Fry, Chinese Beef & 113–14
Vegetables 29, 49
Vegetables, Steamed 137
Vegetables, Summer, Rice with 92–3
Vegetarian Pizza 114–15
Visualising 80–1
Vitamin A 51
Vitamin B complex 25, 35, 51
Vitamin B1 27, 49
Vitamin B2 26, 27, 49
Vitamin B6 27, 49
Vitamin B12 27, 33, 45, 49
Vitamin C 27, 32, 49, 51
Vitamin E 27, 49, 51
Vitamin F 51
Vitamin supplements 26–7, 35, 45, 49–51
Voll, Dr 70

Watercress & Potato Soup 88
Weight loss, avoiding 31
Wheatgerm oil 30
White Sauce 137

Yeast extract 30
Yoga 81–2
Yoghurt 30
Yoghurt, Spicy Chicken in 111
Yoghurt Salsa 93

Zinc 52